RED HOT
MAMAS

RED HOT MAMAS

COMING INTO OUR OWN AT FIFTY

COLETTE DOWLING

BANTAM BOOKS
NEW YORK · TORONTO · LONDON · SYDNEY · AUCKLAND

This edition contains the complete text
of the original hardcover edition.
NOT ONE WORD HAS BEEN OMITTED.

RED HOT MAMAS

A Bantam Book

PUBLISHING HISTORY

Bantam hardcover edition published March 1996
Bantam trade paperback edition / March 1997

ISBN 0-553-37495-8

Published simultaneously in the United States and Canada

Bantam Books are published by Bantam Books, a division of Bantam Dou-
bleday Dell Publishing Group, Inc. Its trademark, consisting of the words
"Bantam Books" and the portrayal of a rooster, is Registered in U.S. Patent
and Trademark Office and in other countries. Marca Registrada. Bantam
Books, 1540 Broadway, New York, New York 10036.

PRINTED IN THE UNITED STATES OF AMERICA

BVG   10 9 8 7 6 5 4 3 2

To my mother, Gladys Stearley Hoppmann, whose richly nuanced conversations with me, in her late eighties, proved that she remains, unquestionably, a Red Hot Mama—as well as my most significant friend and role model.

CONTENTS

ACKNOWLEDGMENTS

I DECIDED TO WRITE a book on midlife women because, in my own life, turning fifty presented challenges I'd never had to face before. I wanted to talk with the women whose work, and whose lives, would give me some understanding of the psychological issues I was facing at this new stage of life.

First—and it was a great place to begin my research—was a brilliant study by Lois W. Banner of how historical attitudes toward sexuality and power in women affect us as we age. *In Full Flower* was eye-opening on the out-and-out hatred of sexuality in older women that percolates beneath the surface of the culture even today—and of what that can do to us.

The physiological status of midlife women—including mood, libido, and the ability to think clearly—is just as important as the psychological to our overall well-being. It is affected far more by hormonal changes than has heretofore been recognized. I thank the many scientists and educators I interviewed whose wonderful research and articulate manner of explaining it allowed me to transform my own health at midlife—and, I hope, write about it in a way that will help others to do the same. Among these are Barbara B. Sherwin, Ph.D., of McGill University, and Philip Sarrel, M.D., Professor of Obstetrics and Gynecology and Psychiatry at the Yale University School of Medicine, both of whom have done ground-breaking research on estrogen's role in the well-being of women in midlife and beyond. Sheryl Sherman, Ph.D., Director of the Aging Institute of the National Institutes of Health, gave me a framework for understanding the vastly important research presented by both basic and social scientists at the institute-sponsored Menopause Workshop, in 1993.

The special challenges to midlife women of being caretakers to both their parents and their children has become grist for the mill of both therapists and social service agencies. Of tremendous help to me in grasping the growing importance of this issue in the lives of women turning fifty was Monica McGoldrick, Director of the Family Institute of New Jersey and associate professor of Clinical Psychiatry at the Robert Wood Johnson Medical School.

Vivian Fenster Ehrlich, Executive Director of DOROT, a social service agency on Manhattan's Upper West Side, helped found the Caregiver's Center, and was generous with her time in talking to me about midlifers' need for help in caring for the older generation.

Carol Anderson, Ph.D., Professor of Psychiatry at the University of Pittsburgh Medical School and Administrator, Western Psychiatric Institute, devotes herself to studying the social and psychological issues of midlife women. I met Carol at a Harvard-sponsored conference for couples therapists, where she spoke about the need for couples in their fifties to reevaluate—and often restructure—their marriages. I have also been influenced by her pioneering ideas on living alone, and how therapists can help women at midlife become comfortable with being single.

Donna Boundy, MSW, gave me a great deal of help in understanding women's psychological resistance, at midlife, to managing their money and investing adequately for the future. She also helped in the computer organization of my research.

Robine Andrau, whose own midlife transition was capped by a degree in library science, helped me gain access to work being done at the Wellesley College Center for Research on Women. Robine also conducted computer searches whose data formed the underpinnings for several chapters of this book.

Rebecca Daniels helped in the interviewing of some of the sixty-five women in their fifties whose stories are the flesh and blood of *Red Hot Mamas*.

Finally, I thank all the courageous women who were willing to put their experiences out there so that others might benefit. Included in this group is Gretchen Cryer, the thoughtful and creative author and star of *I'm Getting My Act Together and Taking It On the Road,* who shared with me the various crises of her fifties decade and how she dealt with them.

Last of all I am grateful to my mother, Gladys Stearley Hoppmann, whose courage and openness in dealing with her eighties has become the major inspiration for my life as I am living it today, in my fifties.

RED HOT
MAMAS

CHAPTER I

THE MAMAS

A GENERATION ARRIVES AT MIDLIFE

Coming Into Our Own • *The Way It Was* • *The Way It Is* •
The Original Red Hot Mamas •
Choice Points: The Revolution Among Midlife Women

IT WAS WILLA'S fiftieth. The women kept surging out onto the floor to dance, while the men stood around the edges of the lofty, cathedral-ceilinged living room and watched. Catherine had made a tape of all those songs from the 1970s, when their lives had begun to change. Tonight, there was something incantatory about the voices, the clapping, the Reeboks and cowboy boots beating rhythmically on the floor. The Mamas, many of them having reached fifty but some still in their forties, were jubilant. The dancing was hot. Claire, visiting from the city and dressed in black biker's shorts, high-tops, and a motor-cycle jacket, was especially fun to watch. Her hair was gray as weath-ered wood, short as a boy's, and her smile was ecstatic. Her body moved as fluidly as if she were much younger, but with this assur-ance, this strength. That combination of social confidence and physi-cal endurance, said Susan, back in the kitchen inhaling guacamole, was killer.

THERE are, for such a small town, a surprising number of us edging up to, or at, or just beyond the age of fifty. For us, this number means something entirely different from what it has in the past, although *what* it means we are not entirely sure. The town is Woodstock. Many of the women here are expatriates of New York who, at one time or another during the last twenty years, left the city and came a hundred miles north, to live in an arts community that was associated with freedom.

It isn't the usual small town. Most of us still have a connection with New York; ex-husbands are there, or grown children, or agents or galleries. The women I know don't relate to being "middle-aged," although they're quite proud of having arrived at fifty. They are bright, brash, irreverent, funny, introspective, neurotic, and caring—and they're out there. It's a new time, a new age, and these are new women. They wear their skirts short, their feet weighted down with Doc Martens. Whether or not they are currently "in a relationship" they feel a connection with their own sexual energy. It's the same thing, my friend Willa says, as creative energy.

I have come to think of these women as the Mamas. They are bursting forth in their lives; they are engaged. Though shaped by the particular choices we've made, the Mamas reflect a generation—millions upon millions in our active and energetic prime who are bringing about a cultural shift. That menopause has come out of the closet is only a part of it. We are the first who came of age with the women's movement to enter this stage of life, and we are doing it—as we've always done everything—differently.

Women entering their fifties today are better educated, more independent, more financially self-sufficient and more involved in community and political life than midlife women have ever been before. We have a chance, now, for a second bloom. It is *our* time, a vivid age when we are freer and more individuated than we were when we were younger. At last we are confident in our strengths, accepting of our limitations, and wise in our ability to adapt, be flexible, dance to the rhythm of our own needs.

But bringing this new chance for growth to fruition is not something that will happen automatically. The second bloom can be cut down, as could the first, by the freak weather of environmental stress, by illness, lack of nurturance, or by a failure of nerve, an inability to seize the moment. To bloom again one needs consciousness, information, perhaps even a sense of mission: I am going to take this decade by its lapels, and—

And *what*? How do we think about the future, how do we plan? What are the limitations, the goals, the possibilities? Could we actually change careers? Enter a new relationship? Pick up and move to Tuscany?

It is different today than it was for past generations of women who, if they were lucky (and how many actually were?) "retired" at midlife. Went out into the garden. Whiled away their afternoons in the sunshine telling stories to their grandchildren. Today—because the life span has opened up—the questions that lie before us at the midlife juncture are new.

What is the most exciting, the most fruitful, and the most organic way to use the next thirty or forty years?

How, where, and in whose company shall we spend them?

And what do we need to do to protect our options and harness our energy?

THE fact is, we are in the middle of a social transition for which there are no guidelines. The first generation who came up with the women's movement to hit fifty, the Mamas are breaking the age barrier. Once again, we're pioneering uncharted territory. We like men, although there are times when we feel closer to women. What we have with our children—those of us who've had them—is open and satisfying. What we have with one another is supportive, empowering us to move out and do more. We feel more connected to more people than perhaps our mothers did at this age. At fifty, we are challenged by a sense of adventure, stimulated by the wit and irony of life. We see the possibilities of this "second half" of adulthood that lies ahead, and we don't back off.

Although, of course, that isn't all there is to it.

COMING INTO OUR OWN

THIS is a generation of women who've made new arrangements with life, who perhaps never married, or have been married and divorced a number of times, or have been separated for so long it feels like divorce. Some of us are already widowed. I was widowed when I was barely forty. At the time, it didn't feel like being widowed since I'd left my husband years earlier and was then, and for some years thereafter, living with someone else. Now, for the first time in my life, I live alone. I have learned to like this very much; still, when asked on some official form to categorize myself I hesitate, unable to choose between Widow and Single. Actually, I like to think that I defy category. In Woodstock, most of us like to think that. Willa, still technically married, has been separated from her second husband for twelve years and remains hopelessly friendly with him. He lives in the same town.

Helen, long divorced—and thus, the forms would have it, Single—refuses to associate herself with any marital state. Fourteen years ago she cut her nails and sold her jewelry to come and live in Woodstock, renting a gatekeeper's house and telling her children they'd better learn to like it. Their father had been building them a big colonial in Great Neck when Helen tired of life with long fingernails and left. In Woodstock she started a bookshop, bought, eventually, a farmhouse, and has had lovers over the years. Now she is with someone new, a man she's been driving up the Thruway to see for over a year, a doctor-turned-sculptor, and they have decided that they will live together. "But I will never again," she says, "make dinner for a man."

The point being that nothing, anymore, is what it would have been in the lives of women our age even twenty years ago. The old categories are gone, and with them, certain expectations. Things have opened up.

There was a moment during a party recently when all the women were in my kitchen at the same time. (Probably it was time to clear the dishes for dessert.) Someone brought up age, and we discovered that the six of us ranged from 49 to 59. For some reason, this made us giddy. Immediately the subject turned to sex—or rather, to our ambivalence about it at this midpoint, when all the talk is of how to stay alive and still have a modicum of fun.

"Did you *see* today's *Woodstock Times*?" asked Fiona.

" 'Caution! Air bubbles break condoms. Smooth out air bubbles as you roll condom onto erect (hard) penis'!" Susan had memorized the article word for word.

We laughed. Among the locals, *The Woodstock Times* is known as the school paper, its coverage limited to the campuslike environment in which, in this small mountain town, we live. The condom article was written to supply certain information to kids that they weren't getting elsewhere and certainly not in school. By afternoon, everyone in Woodstock, regardless of age, gender, or sexual inclination was talking about it.

"I never knew about the air bubbles," said Catherine contemplatively, as if the whole long history of her sex life were passing before her eyes.

"It isn't worth it," said Fiona, standing in the open doorway of the kitchen and holding her cigarette outside. Fiona wonders, sometimes, if she isn't staying in her marriage mostly because of AIDS.

I stacked the dishwasher. Catherine, newly divorced, said these days a lot of people stay married just so they don't have to use condoms.

Susan, whose husband has been known to wander, said maybe that isn't so foolproof. Maybe everyone ought to use condoms, married or not, because who knows what has happened earlier in a person's life? There is such a thing as denial, after all.

Willa says things are too tense to just go out and fool around. Not only is there AIDS to think about, there's age. Does she even have the juice to motivate a search for someone new? "It's like what happens to mortgage money when the market is down," she says.

Things dry up, is what she means.

I tossed in the soap and started the dishwasher. The month was August. The year 1992.

The conversation in my kitchen, on that hot summer night, lasted about twelve minutes and was the most riveting of the evening. Who were we, at this stage of life, where were we going, and what could we expect along the way? When we rejoined our men friends— some gay, some straight, only two of us a part of what by any stan-

dard would be called "a couple"—we felt a letdown. Having left behind the fascinating subject of this uncharted stage in our lives, we
had returned to the dining table, where we sat man-woman, man-
woman, clinging to a comfortable social form, when in fact we were a
new hybrid. Our generation of women had been reared traditionally,
but we were seized, early in our adult lives, with a fierce desire to turn
everything upside down. That desire hasn't left us. Thus, returning to
the men in the dining room felt a little like retreating to the back
ranks after a brief but exhilarating moment on the revolutionary front.
Sex, of course, was only a part of it. (A smaller and smaller part,
according to Catherine.) The fact was, we were having these ex-
changes—in the kitchen, the women's room, at the office water
cooler—because at midlife, we were once again women without
guidelines, braving a new cultural frontier.

The Way It Was

MIDLIFE used to be associated with retirement, that great golden dream
when you got to take off and see what the rest of the country was like.
This was when you and the old man would get up before dawn, and
he would put on his hip-waders and catch the fish, and you would
take out the frying pan and cook them up for breakfast. Now was the
time to enjoy life, to *live*. That's what retirement was, the time when
you finally got to *have* a life. Everything else was supposed to lead up
to that moment with the woodsmoke curling up blue and a whole
lazy day ahead, and you and your husband like some sort of gray-
haired twins, with nothing abrasive left between you, all argument
resolved, money safe, philosophies either entwined or ignored, and if
you were fortunate, a few good tosses in the hay left before it was all
over.

   Now our generation arrives at midlife to find that, thank God, it
isn't going to be like that at all. Of course, the first half of our adult
lives didn't turn out the way it was supposed to, either. We have
always been out of sync with the generation before us. What they told

us would happen, if they told us anything, was almost invariably off the mark.

They told us we'd get married, and have babies, and cast our lot with a workadaddy hero who'd take care of us for the rest of our lives.

Wrong.

They told us we'd "make a home" for our family, but if gathering together bits and pieces from auctions and flea markets, and making the occasional half-a-homemade pie with a frozen Oronoko crust, and letting the kids go to school in the morning with whatever they felt like wearing on their scabby little backs and then holing up on the foam couch with our Pall Malls and our dog-eared copies of *The Golden Notebook* because we always felt so damnably *behind* wasn't making a home, well, we didn't do that either.

The truth is, we spent our lives catching up, making grown-ups of ourselves while they had expected us to remain little girls. We let the housekeeping go to hell and got educated. We refused to play Candyland with the kids because it was too boring, but we did write them stories, and sing to them, slightly weepy ballads from the 1960s. They may have first heard Dylan coming from our sad and disappointed throats as they lay in their rickety bunk beds on colorful weeks-old sheets.

We were women on the cusp of a major change. I can remember my daughter complaining she was the only kid in second grade who had to make her own lunch. By the time these children reached third grade—boom, it was over. They were *all* scooping out the peanut butter from half-gallon jugs, slapping it onto whole-wheat bread, and throwing it into a brown paper lunch bag before going to school in the morning.

Our mothers, in the meantime, wanted to know how we justified the dust balls floating listlessly around the books stacked by our beds (*The Women's Room, Fear of Flying, Diary of a Mad Housewife*). What were we going to *do*, they asked; how were we going to get out of this rut? Seeing that we were not on the same paths they were, our mothers assumed we were in a rut. They worked hard to get us on the right track. My mother once bought a trowel and a can of ready-mixed cement and tried to smooth off the windowsills in my apartment, thinking it would be easier for me to clean them if they weren't splintered and rough. I was not a particularly clean daughter. Oh, I hauled out my vacuum every few weeks, whenever I had a free moment, but windowsills, rough or smooth, were never high on my agenda.

My friends were pretty much the same. Still, it isn't as if we were goofing off. We were *changing,* whether or not our mothers knew or accepted it, and change takes energy. Eventually we went back to school or we went to work. Many of us ended up doing both. Those of us who hadn't finished college before the babies started coming finished when the kids went to school. Those of us who'd gotten B.A.'s decided to go back. There are more M.A.'s and M.B.A.'s and Ph.D.'s in our generation of women than in any generation before. We got jobs and made moves. Many of us left our husbands. We joined support groups, did consciousness-raising, became survivors. We read *The Joy of Sex* and compared notes with our friends on park benches in the playground. We ordered vibrators from mail-order catalogs. We were like schoolgirls let loose in the big city for the first time.

Not to say that it wasn't hard. Family life was tenuous. There was lots of therapy and not nearly enough money to go around. At times, our kids would still be waiting in front of school at four o'clock because someone had screwed up and forgotten to go get them. But here's the important thing: We got free. We bloomed. And we had the good fortune to know we were blooming. It was a kind of meta-experience: We bloomed, and we saw ourselves blooming, and we saw our friends blooming, and we saw Gloria, and Betty, and Robin and all those *Ms.* people putting out that magazine with gritty pictures of women, black and white, and we *congratulated* ourselves. You don't do that unless you're feeling empowered, and there was no doubt that we were. We had changed things for women, for ourselves, radically.

Then came a new decade, another shift. We turned forty. Many of us remarried, and some eventually left these husbands, too. Some—they're the unusual ones now—stayed with the same man for the duration.

Others never married at all.

Still others hooked up with women. Our generation did everything differently, and we turned our lives upside down. We had money of our own, and Lord knows we spent it. We lost fat and built

lean muscle. We organized and took political st⟨
denly . . .

Suddenly we were fifty—the first generat⟨.
this age and conceive of ourselves as free. The first tɔ
our disposal, the first to have choices. Today women at fifty cₐ⟨
what their next thirty years will be. Instead of seeing fifty as the begiₙ
ning of the end, as earlier generations of women did, we see it as a
new beginning.

And yet we feel vulnerable.

THE WAY IT IS

BECAUSE no previous generation of midlife women had the luxury of
seeing decades of productive time roll out before them, we who came
of age with the women's movement are in the position, once again, of
having to do it for the first time. Fifty is a watershed year, when we
sense that we could slip down either the left bank or the right. If we
retreat from the challenges ahead, we will *not* start a new business,
begin a directing career, move to a different city. Unless we take action, we will likely miss out on the new joys available to us, the
chance to toughen our minds, express ourselves fearlessly, become the
feisty, political, and argumentative beings we may have repressed
when we were younger.

When I began talking, at Willa's party, with Claire of the biker
shorts, I found out that, spunky appearance to the contrary, her life
was far from under control. She had recently returned to the States
after a thirteen-year stint, postdivorce, in Saint John's, and life, suddenly, had turned tumultuous. She'd lost her restaurant on the island
during the recession and had had to declare bankruptcy. At about that
time, her two daughters left home, one for a job in California, one for
graduate school in New York. Suddenly, the abyss. Claire had an idea
she wanted to find work as a chef, but she kept vacillating, afraid to
plunge in for fear of another failure. Part of the time she lived with a
friend; the rest of the time she squeezed into a one-room walk-up in

enwich Village with her daughter. New York wasn't what it had een when she'd left. Now, without a real home, and with her kids flying off to the four corners of the earth, Claire felt painfully dislocated.

A bankruptcy and the change from island life to urban hell, topped off by kids moving out into lives of their own, may seem dramatic, but Claire's losses reflect the experience of many women in their fifties: The changes can pile up so fast we have a hard time integrating them. When Claire's sense of herself began to unravel in Saint John's, she decided to return to the town where she'd grown up. But when she got there, the reality was not very nurturing. At 51, she was divorced, jobless, and female in the most competitive city in the world. For the first time she felt handicapped by her age. "I'm a chef with a lot of experience, but I walk into these places, and they actually say to me, 'We only hire younger women.' "

THE fact of aging, the possibility of illness, the onset of limitations—all of this has become vividly real. Yet there is an up side to recognizing that life doesn't go on forever. Fifty is a jumping-off time. It may not be a midlife identity crisis, as social scientists thought of it in the 1950s and 1960s. One of the great joys of arriving at midlife is that one's sense of self is already in place. But fifty nevertheless has an urgency, a feeling of challenges to be hurdled, and maybe even drastic steps that need to be taken. We get this now-or-never feeling. We want to make it *happen*.

And to do that, we have to take chances.

At fifty, I left a relationship that hadn't been working for a long time. We had been together for sixteen years. "The irony," my partner said, "is that of the two of us, you turned out to be the less dependent one." He had been wanting the separation as much as I, but he might have hung on indefinitely, he said, because it seemed easier.

For me, the presumed safety of staying together had become more confining than comforting. At the same time, what a risk it would be to leave! I had never been alone before, not really. When I separated from my husband twenty years earlier, I had had three young children in tow, and while I certainly knew loneliness, I didn't know what it was to actually *be* alone—empty house in the morning, empty house at night. Now I would find out.

And there would be other things, events that pile up like waves rolling onto you before you can catch your breath. At 26, my oldest child would be stricken with a serious depression and would need my help as she put her life back together again. My mother, the healthy, hardy farm girl from Nebraska, would contract a rare blood disease that left her vulnerable to every conceivable infection. My 84-year-old father would spend ten tragic weeks in the hospital fighting to recover from a car accident before he finally succumbed.

From this point on, our parents' lives will be increasingly riddled with illnesses and setbacks. And so it seems that just as we are ready to let loose, perhaps for the first time in our lives, we are paradoxically faceup against the hardest thing of all: The gut-level acknowledgment of mortality—our parents', and our own.

WHILE all this is happening, so, of course, is menopause. The hormone changes that accompany it affect us in many ways. For months and months, without knowing why, I became hoarse, exhausted, and prone to bouts of severe perimenopausal bleeding. The doctors took an unconscionably long time to figure out that the bleeding had made me anemic, and that—possibly in conjunction with the anemia—my thyroid wasn't functioning adequately. Depression, with these conditions, is unavoidable.

Inevitably, perhaps, I developed money problems. Somehow during these years, I didn't acknowledge that my income was lower than it had been, and that my expenses, now that I was living alone, were higher. I began to do the unthinkable—dip early into my retirement fund.

In all, the beginning of my fifties decade was a whirlwind of change, loss, and growth. I knew that my experience wasn't unique, but often I felt confused and alone. What *is* this? I began to wonder. Help! Somebody throw me a lifeline!

My lifeline came in the form of a therapist named Beveraly, and from my decision to write this book. Beveraly helped me reconstruct the past and open myself to what my needs are now. Writing has helped me to connect to the midlife challenges others are experiencing. More and more, I turn to women for succor and guidance, for their special humor and down-to-earth willingness to look life in the eye. And so, with tape recorder in hand, I visited with dozens of women around the country, some sixty-five in all, who were in the thick of it. My intent was not to do a survey, in the social science sense, but to ask and listen, as a journalist does, to the voices of my generation. I wanted to learn of the journeys these women were taking, and I wanted to record them in their own words as they break new ground. They are part of a new breed, women who at midlife are in touch with being sexual, energetic, and powerful. Women who are facing new choices and finding new places to take their lives.

One woman I interviewed decided to take hospice training, not because she had a terminally ill loved one, but because she felt cut off from her own mortality.

Another told me she had never done the "hard work" of developing her mind and wanted to do it now, "while I still have a mind." At 49, not long after I interviewed her, she began work on a novel, having never written before.

Yet another woman felt herself, at fifty, to be stepping off the edge of an old map. Esther had spent most of her life cleaning houses for others, and now she'd left an abusive husband, gotten a better-paying job in a hospital, and taken an apartment of her own. We sat together in a small park in Saugerties, New York, one bright spring morning, and she said, astonished, "I'm fifty years old and I don't know who I am."

The important thing was that she'd courageously carved out a space where she could begin to find out.

I was fascinated by how the women I interviewed were making meaning of the midlife transition, and the wit, wisdom, and inventiveness with which they met their challenges. At fifty, their lives were stunningly complicated—rich, painful, joyful, and sometimes frightening. Listening to their voices later on the tape deck in my car, I began to feel myself a part of this great generation of women once again.

I wanted to name this new experience we are having, and to offer new, more positive images, with which, at this stage, we might identify. Early in my research I had heard about support groups popping up in California for women this age that were calling themselves Red Hot Mamas. Whenever I mentioned this, in the lectures I give, women would cheer. The phrase captured something we all felt: It isn't over yet—not by a long shot.

At about this time, I read a book on women, aging, and power. In *In Full Flower,* University of Southern California historian Lois Banner tells of the respect black culture pays its midlife and older women, who it thinks of as "mamas." The denigration of aging women so prevalent in white American culture doesn't happen in black culture, says Banner. "Among blacks, aging women are valued."

Valued, they are perceived not as over the hill but as active, forceful members of society, equipped to bring about change.

And as they have been perceived, so they have behaved.

THE ORIGINAL RED HOT MAMAS

"IN every southwest Georgia county," wrote a student organizer in the 1960s, "there is always a 'mama.' "

A mama was a militant member of the black community, outspoken, understanding, "and willing to catch hell, having already caught her share." Respected for her age and experience, and crucial to organizing the black community in northern urban ghettoes as well as southern rural hamlets, the mama assumed leadership in overturning white patriarchy.

Earlier in this century, when the blues were gaining strength as a musical idiom, feisty black female vocalists became extremely popular. No matter that these women were aging, overweight, or showing on their faces the experience of their years. "They dressed and lived in high style," writes Banner, "and the black community called them 'goddesses' and 'high priestesses.' " From their energetic style, and from the lusty, self-validating lyrics of the jazz singers among them, came the term *red hot mama.*

Do we have red hot mamas today? We have, certainly, the wonderful Etta James. In nascent form, we have nervy Queen Latifah.

(Imagine her at fifty!) But perhaps most notably—her story has become one of triumph for women around the world—we have Tina Turner, who, at 53, was dubbed by writer Maureen Orth "the queen mother of rock 'n' roll."

Reporting on a Carnegie Hall performance in the spring of 1993, Orth described Turner's tight black leather catsuit with tails and high platform boots. "Her hair (piece) was a flying wedge of layered copper, and her powerful voice pierced the darkness like lightning: 'When I was a little girl . . . I had a rag doll.'" As she bounced about the stage with her little Pony steps, "those trademark legs swathed in leather," the energy she'd displayed at the beginning of her career, twenty-seven years earlier, was as electrifying as ever. That's Red Hot Mama energy, and while it includes sexuality, it is not merely sexual. It has to do with the integrity, aggressiveness, and self-affirmation of women who are able, at midlife, to respect themselves. It has to do with their capacity—which often doesn't arrive until now—to be *among* women, to feel validated by them rather than competitive with them.

As anyone knows who saw *What's Love Got to Do With It?*, the film based on Tina's life, her years with Ike—when he thought *he* was the one with the talent, that *he* was running the show—were horrible. "The mouth was always distorted, the eyes were always black," Tina told Orth in her dressing room after the performance. Kneeling on the sofa, clutching a pillow, Turner pointed out the old scars. "When she pushes up the bangs of her wig," Orth observed, "you can see a tiny part of her fuzzy white hairline."

Somehow it was shocking, this sexual cannonball hiding bone-white hair.

Or was the reverse what was shocking—that someone with that hair could have such energy, such legs, such unmitigated verve?

IN the chapters to follow you will find a group of women I call "the Mamas" appearing throughout. They are fictionalized portraits representing the core group of "girlfriends" on whom most of us, as we age, come increasingly to rely. These women challenge us, mother us. They become our Greek chorus. They watch the revolution going on in our lives and offer comment. They validate and mirror us. They cheer us on.

In addition to the Mamas' are stories of women I talked to around the country. To protect anonymity, I have given them changed first names (and no last names) and altered certain details. The rest is as it comes off the tape recorder. The voices, and the women, are real.

CHOICE POINTS: THE REVOLUTION AMONG MIDLIFE WOMEN

"FOR women who have awakened to new possibilities in middle age, or who were born into the current women's movement and have escaped the usual rhythms of the once traditional female existence," says Carolyn Heilbrun, "the last third of life is likely to require new attitudes and new courage."

I came to understand, as I worked my way through my fifties decade, that for women today, midlife presents all the challenge and opportunity—and all the potential tumult—that we experienced at adolescence. Those wild, unknown possibilities we apprehended at sixteen, that unique mixture of fear and excitement, is here again. Much as we had to put childhood behind us then, we have to put early adulthood behind us now. Much as we took the leap and embraced the future then, so we have to take the leap now.

The way it felt to me, as I entered my fifties, was that I needed to put myself in a new place. It wasn't a question, this time, of getting out of a marriage, or finding a new love, or going back to school. It was more a matter of redefining myself, of digging deep into my character to discover what was most real, most enduring—and of constructing my life in a way that would give prominence to that deeper sense of self, that would let it shine.

But how? How to do that? Nothing I'd been through in the past seemed to address this need to be in touch with my deepest self. There was no program, no specific course that in and of itself would take me to the untried parts of myself that were now yearning to be expressed. If I wanted to get to this new place, I would have to open up, reach out, trust.

Much would have to change. Ultimately, I would give up the family homestead. I would leave old friends and make new ones. I would change, and in the process I would discover what type of day I needed to sustain me, what type of air and light, what sounds. Without the old insecurities holding me back, I would grow and flourish in my prime, would feel that I had come home to myself at last.

But in the course of what essentially would become a spiritual journey, a quest for deepening, practical issues needed to be addressed. In talking with other women my age I heard the same issues come up again and again. And after several years of research, in which I spoke, as well, to therapists and social scientists, I began to be able to extract a kind of schema for confronting the obstacles that can prevent us from coming into our own at fifty.

There are eight important issues that require attention from us at this stage. I decided to call them Choice Points. There are moments in time when we take actions, or don't take them, and the decisions we make at these moments profoundly change the way our lives spin out. The chapters in this book are devoted to the eight Choice Points that I believe will play the most significant role in determining the quality of our lives in the next thirty years. Virtually all of them stem from the complexities of contemporary life—the brand-new social and psychological situations in which women of this age are finding themselves today.

The first Choice Point addresses the fact that there are social barriers to women's aging happily and productively—namely, the double whammy of sexism and ageism that hits women at midlife. It is possible to assert ourselves against these barriers, to choose *not* to go along with traditional views of what's "appropriate" for women our age. Instead, we can join our sisters, some of whose stories are told in Chapter II ("What's Age Got to Do With It?"), in defining a new midlife reality—a task that requires courage and creativity.

There are times when the caretaking burdens of midlife seem overwhelming, and we resent them, wondering, Where is all this freedom everyone's always talking about? There is fresh potential, at this age, for becoming swamped with responsibilities—the Woman-in-the-Middle phenomenon, whereby we are bookended by the needs of both the younger generation and the older. Because of our conditioning, and because of society's persistent expectation that *women* are the ones responsible for the well-being of family members, we risk losing new opportunities to the burdens of caretaking. Again, there is a choice to be made. Chapter III, "Caught in the Middle," tells of women inventing new ways to be available to loved ones, while not losing their own chances for growth and development.

How we feel about aging has a lot to do with messages we've taken inside ourselves—"internalized," as psychologists call the process. Insidious because it's largely unconscious, internalization imprints us with messages that linger within, long after outer circumstances have changed. We're left with a conflict between the inner and the outer. For the midlife woman, that can translate into "Fifty is a gorgeous, free, transcendent age. I'm *thrilled* to be fifty!" But also: "I hate being fifty. I hate losing my looks, I hate thinking about the foreshortening of time." Feeling torn, we may temporize, tread water, let these potentially productive years drift by out of focus, without taking the steps necessary for making this stage of life *happen*. Another Choice Point, here. As explored in Chapter IV, ("This Is What Fifty Looks Like"), we can confront the stereotypes that in the past have hampered women from realizing new agendas as they grow older. But we have to be aware of them, and where they come from. Many of the negative images of midlife women derive from society's fear of the sexual energy and greater sexual freedom of women after menopause. As recently as the Fifties, Sixties, and Seventies, older women who liked sex were considered pathological. Today's midlife women still suffer from negative images of older women and it is up to us to change them—to make that choice.

It's part of society's myth that if we're not in a marriage, we're alone. That idea is changing. Still, for those of us who were married for years, finding happiness in the single state will require something more than passivity. It will mean constructing social networks, finding intellectual challenges, perhaps even creating new values—developing a whole new sense of what is important in life. Many of us are alone now for the first time. Others are finding that intimate relations with husbands, partners, and friends require redefinition. The fourth

Choice Point deals with these issues of intimacy. How we choose to be in our intimate relationships will affect the quality of our lives, from here on out, more profoundly than ever.

And what of the loss of our sex hormones? Women cry over the unbidden changes of midlife. We cry when our hearing dims and our memory needs constant jogging, even though we are told this may be merely "hormonal," and likely will pass. We watch youth fade—sometimes, if hysterectomy is involved, with appalling suddenness—and we weep in secret, for there is no open acknowledgment of these losses and of what they mean to us. Physical well-being, for women, is complicated at midlife by hormonal changes. The fifth Choice Point involves making the decision to educate ourselves, to keep up with the rapidly emerging information on sex hormones and their effects on brain, behavior, mood, and memory. Chapter VI, "Hormone Wars," shows how the competing interests of science and feminism can obstruct our getting important information, and properly interpreting what we do get. The Choice Point, here, is acquiring health information in every way that we can, and developing our own ways of using it.

Choice Point Six involves facing the sexual changes that occur in men and women at midlife. Although sexuality doesn't die off as we age, it certainly changes. Knowing what to expect can protect us from disappointment, and from backing off from sex because we're embarrassed by what's happening to us. Midlife sex can actually be freer, more tender, more inventive, and more emotionally satisfying than sex was when we were younger—but to reap these gains, we have to change our attitudes about sex.

The seventh Choice Point has to do with gaining control of money. If midlife women don't start creating financial security for themselves now, they're setting themselves up for decades of late-life purgatory. But women of our generation still experience barriers to taking responsibility for their financial future. Of the sixty-five women I interviewed, only two were investing adequately for retirement, even though some were earning $100,000 a year or more! Chapter VIII, "Money of One's Own," discusses the psychological—and social— barriers to financial independence, and shows us midlife women who are confronting them.

Finally there is the challenge, simply, to move ahead in spite of concerns that we lack the energy and creativity. In spite of our fears of the unknown. Choice Point Eight is about taking the risks required to swing past the frontiers of fifty and into a productive, satisfying mid-life.

Women who learn to adapt, to both create opportunities and accept limitations in order to have a better quality of life, women who make the choices that will allow them to spend more time doing what they want to do, who have a game plan, or goal, will have a better prime. But we may find ourselves losing the game plan when we are in transition, when our children are gone, and perhaps our husbands or partners as well, when we sense both the possibility of greater freedom and a frightening awareness that the only person we can rely on now is *us*.

We have no role models for what's required of us now, no guidelines. But when we share our experiences with one another, we can have, at fifty, the possibility of joy, and of taking off anew. I invite you to enter the lives of these women, to hear their stories, weep for their losses, and be guided by their wisdom.

And I share my own story.

Together we can explore this transition and celebrate its freedom, as we celebrated freedom when the women's movement first took off, and we with it.

CHAPTER II

WHAT'S AGE GOT TO DO WITH IT?

*Breaking the "Stage" Barrier • "Middle Age": The Way It Was •
Transcending Age Consciousness • Taking Up Where the Girl Left Off*

WE ARE DRIVING up the mountain with the sunroof thrown back. Willa, peering into the rearview, is watching in horror as the wind riffles her hair and the white shows. "This is how I'm going to end up getting killed," she says, "checking my roots at sixty miles an hour."

I know women who've taken up motorcycle riding, or rock climbing, or Rollerblading in their fifties. The less adventurous buy convertibles—Miatas, MGs, Mustangs. Those exuberant women you see flying around in scarves and sunglasses, hugging the curves, digging the sensation of going fast, aren't seventeen. They're likely fifty, or sixty, or even seventy. My neighbor Nancy, up the road, streaks down our hill every morning in her silver Miata. Susan has a little yellow CRX with an adorable turned-up butt. Bobbie's kids gave her a red Mustang for her sixtieth, and she drives it in all but the iciest weather.

At first I thought it was compensatory. You lose your sex hormones and start driving a sports car. I'd managed to content myself with an old SAAB whose once-glossy coat grew duller each year. I liked it in spite of its shabbiness. The car functioned like an extension of my body. I drove it one-handed, taking the mountains of Woodstock with my left hand on the wheel, my right gripping a container of coffee. I felt as if I could go to my grave in this car, which knew my wishes almost before I gave the commands.

But then, in my middle fifties, I began getting the urge. For pennies, Fiona had gotten herself an old MG, and for not much more, she'd had it restored and painted British-racing-car green. Mornings, she'd zip past my house, peeling as she took the bend in the road. I began thinking about that car, obsessing on it the way a teenage boy might.

Women entering midlife have few rites of passage, little that acknowledges our new power and freedom, that lets us put it out there and say, "I am viable. I am self-determining and sexy. I treat myself well." Sports cars and motorcycles say that to the world. They say, "I don't sit around, I move. There has been a hurdle, and I have gotten over it and am now on the other side, swinging ahead with my life, grooving on a good set of tires and substantial shocks. I still take risks, but they are calculated, rooted in wisdom and experience."

They say, "This is fun!"

For women at midlife, having a hot car can represent the thrill of release. No more hauling groceries and kids and insufferably dependent Great Danes in the backseat. We're free! We can blare Mitch Ryder and the Detroit Wheels over the Xenon speakers, our platformed high-tops pressing the accelerator as "Devil with the Blue Dress On" shakes the windshield. We can take off from the city at midnight, and cruise up the pitch-black Thruway, cellular phone at the ready, arriving back in Woodstock so late nothing but the stars are out.

ALTERING the picture dramatically for women who are in or about to enter their fifties is the longevity revolution. With people living healthily for decades longer, those of us who are currently in midlife have more productive time ahead than we ever thought we'd have. "It is a phenomenon truly unprecedented in human history," says social psychologist Lydia Bronte. "The longevity revolution took us by surprise. We didn't expect it. We didn't lay any plans for it; no one did anything deliberate to create it. We didn't even realize that such a thing was possible until it happened."

Since the early part of the century, the length of time humans spend in adulthood has more than doubled. That's a greater increase than occurred over the previous two thousand years. In a very brief period of time, thus, women who've arrived at midlife find themselves facing a whole new set of expectations. There are more years of work ahead, requiring us to extend our careers or forge brand-new ones. We will need more money than we had thought to support ourselves in our later years. We will have more prolonged involvement with, and caretaking of, the generation ahead of us. We will have little choice but to prime the physical pump—our bodies—to work better longer.

And of course we will have decisions to make—Choice Points that will mightily affect how good we feel and how productive we can be in these longer lives.

Experts say the new years come not at the end of the life span but at its middle. What we have to contemplate, as Lydia Bronte sees it, is a long *second* middle age (from 50 to 75), following a first middle age that occurs between 35 and 50. Age experts differ on the parameters of the new life span. Walter Bortz II, M.D., an authority on aging at the Stanford University Medical School, describes us as being young until we're 40, middle-aged between 40 and 80, and old from 80 to 120. But whatever numbers we put to it, this newly extended arc of vitality requires us to think differently about our lives. As Bronte, a former director of the Aging Society Project at the Carnegie Corporation, observes, if you're unaware of the longevity factor, "you could reach fifty and think your most creative or productive years are behind you (they aren't); or you could think that you'll be old at sixty-five (you probably won't be)."

Since adult life in women currently lasts about sixty years—from 21 to 81—midadulthood, for us, begins at about fifty. What this means is new opportunity but also untried experiences. The way our parents went through their forties, fifties, and sixties will have little bearing on the way we do. Fifty is not the beginning of "the golden years," as this time of life used to be called, but something quite different. Due to medical advances, we have better health and more energy with which to enjoy our extended midlife.

Still, there are psychological adjustments to be made. Many of us are trying to figure out how to integrate our new second adulthoods with the very different sense we grew up with of how this time of life was supposed to unfold. And the experience is going to be different for women than for men. The radical social and economic changes of the last quarter-century have created for midlife women a new mesa—a place we haven't been before. The emerging understanding of hormones, hot flashes, and postmenopausal sex is only part of it. This may be the first time when women of our generation have felt truly free—free to accomplish, free to choose what's most meaningful for us, free to be powerful. At midlife, a dynamic new aspect of ourselves has a chance to emerge: a go-getter unafraid of her power at last. A dreamer. A creator. There are new levels of emotional and intellectual development to be pursued—a windfall of possibility.

But in speaking with women around the country, I've learned that the challenge to reinvent ourselves at midlife often requires struggle. We need to reshape our identities as persons whose value has to do with a great deal more than the ability to make babies.

BREAKING THE "STAGE" BARRIER

"MIDDLE age" used to be considered the beginning of the end for women, who unlike men were thought to begin losing their appeal the day they turned 45. Sex, adventure, and challenge were expected to throttle fast backward, while the future collapsed into an image of lumpy chenille bathrobes and iron-gray pincurls.

Not that women had a monopoly on midlife *angst*. Debilitating changes were everyone's due. Basically, adults of both genders were pictured as passing overnight from vigor to decline. But with women it happened earlier. Women were thought to be stricken by loss of hormones at about fifty; men, by loss of job identity when they retired at 65. Because society took a dire view of menopause (and lacked information about male hormonal changes), men were thought to have an extra fifteen years or so of vim and vigor before their memories, too, lagged, their joints stiffened, and their brain cells stopped communicating. Eventually we all ended up in the stagnant wasteland called "middle age."

Onto this bleak view of adult development, a provocative new model was subsequently superimposed. One didn't simply fossilize at 45—one could continue to develop, evolving into higher and ever more individuated stages of humanity as the years passed. Erik Erikson, the influential psychoanalyst of the 1940s and 1950s, propounded the idea that adult life consisted of fixed, sequential stages, each of which was to be "mastered." "Stage theory," as it came to be known, offered the comforting idea that growing old follows an immutable pattern. Death might not be kind, but at least the years leading up to it held few surprises. The decline our grandparents faced our parents, too, would have to grapple with, and so, in the same way, would we. The process of aging was presumed to be relentlessly the same for everyone.

"Stages" of life, of course, are social inventions. Childhood wasn't even identified as a separate stage until the eighteenth century. Adolescence was invented in the late nineteenth century, and "youth" and "middle age" emerged in the twentieth. The latest delineation—a distinction without a difference, a lawyer might say—is between the "young-old" and the "old-old." The longer we humans live, apparently, the more stages we require as a way of codifying our life experience, making it more comfortingly predictable than it really is.

In the 1970s, Daniel Levinson elaborated on Erikson's theory, placing specific accomplishments—actually, *male* accomplishments—on the path of adult life considered "normal." A man in his twenties was supposed to marry and begin a career. In his thirties, he would establish himself professionally and solidify his marriage. By the time he reached his forties, he would reassess his commitments and wrench free of his old mentors. This last was known as the BOOM phenomenon: Becoming One's Own Man. BOOM was thought to require a midlife crisis, during which one's outer life and one's inner self-concept underwent a profound change. If a man didn't confront his midlife crisis, he stayed at wimp level, never quite making it to full-blown masculine status.

Picasso comes to mind as a shining example of someone who BOOMed, remaining forever creative, sexual, and sinewy. At 75, Picasso was still a fun guy. His talent for living in his later years, stage theory implied, was no exception to the rule; anyone with courage could fight the good fight of adult development and keep on flying.

Ideally, the end of life brought "integrity," as Erikson called it—psychological integration. Reaching this stage meant being able to accept the whole of one's life for what it was, without any sense of having lost something important along the way. Going hand in hand with integrity was "generativity," a stage when contributing in a lasting way to others became the major occupation. Erikson saw generativity as a trade-off for the loss of youthful vigor.

Certainly this idea that adults develop in much the way that children do was compelling. It implied predictability; it rallied us onward and upward. "One appeal of stage theory was that it outlined spiraling progressions of *improvement*," psychologist Carol Ryff wrote in *Gender and the Life Course*. As they went from stage to stage, people could count on having to confront a clear-cut series of "crises." If they transcended these crises, they could expect to progress to ever higher levels of functioning. Stage theory offered ripe plums to the upwardly mobile. As Gail Sheehy presented it in *Passages,* you couldn't get to Step Two, the "Catch Thirties" decade, unless you first hurdled the developmental tasks of Step One, the "Trying Twenties." It was kind of like school.

In rendering Levinson's theory palatable for the masses, Sheehy offered readers an irresistible theme. So long as they knew what was coming from one decade to the next, and had a modicum of guts, they could step crablike through the minefield of possibilities and come out ahead. *Passages,* at bottom, was about winning—winning the game of adult life.

In 1976, the same year Sheehy's book hit the best-seller list, social scientists began complaining about "pop culture renderings" of life stages. Suddenly the new field of adult development was "in danger," the noted age theorist Orville Brim warned. The public was swallowing the idea of predictable adult stages, he feared, the same way "it seizes on astrology and tea-leaf readings."

As for the catchy notion of a "midlife crisis," the granddaddy of stage theorists, Erik Erikson, had never even used the term. Could it be that adult life involved events and feelings and processes more complicated than the neat schema implied in stage theory?

*   *   *

FEMINIST social scientists played an important role in loosening the grip of stage theorists on adult development. Grace Baruch and Rosalind Barnett, scholars at the Wellesley College Center for Research on Women, found so much variation in the lives of women between 35 and 55 they proposed abandoning any lockstep idea of adult development. In *Lifeprints: New Patterns of Love and Work for Today's Women*, published in 1983, Baruch and Barnett said that stage theory didn't reflect the lives of women, who rarely follow the same life schedules men do. Instead of reassessing their career commitments at forty, for example, some women are only just beginning to make them.

Other women reverse that agenda, making their first commitments to family and children in their forties and even their fifties. For women, Baruch and Barnett point out, "generativity," that presumed pinnacle of maturity, is not a late-life phenomenon at all but something with which they are involved, hands-on, from the time their children are born.

Of course, not all women have children, and that obvious point eventually helped provoke a major shift in the thinking of social theorists, which in turn has contributed to a major opening up of the options available to women. Remarkably, these options continue to open as our lives grow longer.

IN the 1940s, 1950s, and 1960s, marriage was construed as *the* major turning point for women. For us (not for men), choosing a mate was considered the final step in resolving our identity. "The stage of life crucial for the emergence of an integrated female identity is the step from youth to maturity, the stage when the young woman, whatever her career, relinquishes the care received from the parental family in order to commit herself to the love of a stranger and to the care to be given to their offspring," proclaimed Erikson in 1968, putting the final stamp of approval on a theory that was about to crumble. Even as Erikson made his pronouncement, students were barricading college administration offices, half a million of the politically aware were camping in the mud at the Woodstock Festival, and feminists were writing treatises on the politics of orgasm. Nonetheless, an entire generation of psychologists and sociologists took their definition of "normal" female development from Erikson. Even in the 1970s, a woman hoping to "take the step from youth to maturity" was encouraged to believe that "committing herself to the love of a stranger" was the only way to go.

In a few short years, society has moved from one model of adulthood to a very different one—from a short-term model based on a set of predictable stages, to a long-term model with no fixed stages, one that's based on continuous growth and evolution. Moreover, marrying is no longer considered the milestone of female development that it once was. The net of normality has widened to include all sorts of choices and lifestyles. What social scientists are exploring now is how women's lives really unfold—how we actually think and feel about ourselves and our lives from decade to decade, experience to experience, decision to decision.

Both men and women reaching midlife today will likely need to think about their goals and options all over again. But women, for a number of reasons, may find the midlife challenge more complex, and more anxiety-producing, than men do. We expect—and are expected—to earn more money, travel, develop further intellectually, and be open to sex, romance, and new friendships. But we are also expected (as we shall see in Chapter III) to continue being the main caretakers in the family. Wedged between our parents' generation, which is living into its nineties, and our children's generation, which requires help from us into its thirties, we are very much "caught in the middle." Only with conscious planning can we prevent ourselves from being sucked into a vortex of family demands that could keep us from realizing our midlife potential.

"MIDDLE AGE": THE WAY IT WAS

BERNICE Neugarten, an influential researcher in the field of adult development and aging, has written that most people who've reached forty, fifty, or sixty wouldn't want to be young again. But others, including the noted feminist sociologist Alice Rossi, have shown that equanimity about aging depends upon a host of conditions, not the least being financial security and a manageable amount of stress. Feeling good about oneself at midlife, Rossi concludes, is a happy state that befalls women who have had higher education, feel competent in their family roles, and have a high work drive, help from their children, and plenty of social activity outside the home. This doesn't mean that only the privileged are happy, but it does suggest the importance of financial security.

In her 1978 study of women from two small towns in western Massachusetts, Rossi found that those women who *didn't* feel young at fifty were likely to be in stressful marriages. Their lives weren't gratifying enough and they were worriers. Rossi's old-at-fifty subjects were obsessively concerned with their husbands and children, were less likely to feel committed to work (if they worked outside the home at all), and involved themselves in fewer social and cultural activities than those who felt younger at midlife.

Rossi broke her sample into two groups: younger mothers who were 36 to 43, and older mothers who were 45 to 51. *Most* women in both groups, she found, yearned to be younger. In fact, the older they were, the younger they fantasized being. Asked what age they'd pick to be if they could be any age they wanted, *half the women wanted to be under thirty.* Those who were in their forties wanted to be eight years younger, on average. Those in their fifties wanted to be fifteen years younger!

Rossi thinks their fantasies of being younger had to do with wishing to escape their feelings of bleakness about their current lives. (Of the 68 women in the study, two-thirds were employed, and one in five was going to school. A third hadn't gone past high school.) While the younger women were aware of early signs of aging—less agility, not snapping back as quickly from late hours, difficulty keeping weight down—the older women responded on a deeper level, says Rossi, "often with a note of despair."

In these two Massachusetts towns in the 1970s, the forty-year-old women were *out* there—active, having fun, living their lives. But by 48, things were tougher. By that time they felt mired in family responsibility. Worrying about suicidal mothers and fathers going into nursing homes, and about children with financial and drug problems, they were being throttled by the "sandwich generation" squeeze. And they showed many symptoms of depression, including a lack of optimism about the future.

Not surprisingly, the women who reported the most stress also indicated "shorter life preferences." Those who imagined themselves dying sooner were the ones who wished they were much younger. "Middle-aged mothers who look longingly in the direction of youth or darkly ahead to a premature death," Rossi stated, did so *not* because they'd internalized the culture's glorification of youth *but because their lives were too stressful.* In their fantasies, they wanted out—either by being younger or by not living much longer. Some actually said they would rather die young than have to experience becoming old!

A fairly high percentage of women in this 1978 study, it's important to note, were on the low end economically. A third of them had family incomes below $15,000. In other studies, Rossi found money to be a *major* factor in determining the equanimity with which people age. The more money we have, the less disturbing growing older seems to be.

In the 1970s, when Rossi was conducting her study, society's new attitudes toward midlife were only just beginning to emerge. Midlife itself had hardly begun to change. Today, with better health, education, and financial status than women have ever enjoyed, those approaching midlife have new worlds of opportunity and experience ahead of them. We don't have to look back, wishing we were younger, because we've so much to look forward to.

TRANSCENDING AGE CONSCIOUSNESS

"THE good thing," Helen was saying, "is that no matter how old we get, we'll always be able to dance to King Creole and the Coconuts."

She was referring to the fact that she'd just gotten a gold card from her health club in honor of five straight years of membership. It conferred on her a five percent break on club fees—unnervingly close, she thought, to a senior citizen's discount.

But the fact was, she was fit. She didn't look "her age." She didn't feel "her age." *Was* she, even, "her age"?

Or as Willa sums up, "What's age got to do with it?"

We may be Red Hot Mamas, but because this version of midlife we're experiencing is so new, we can still hold ourselves back with concerns about what's "age-appropriate." Sometimes we worry whether we're "too old" to be going back to school, learning flamenco, comparing properties of different types of condoms. Part of our anxiety comes from the fact that we have no models that explain or validate our lives right now.

After her divorce, Marilyn Mason went through a period when she was dating at the same time her kids were, worrying about their birth control practices as she worried about her own. And she was besieged by doubts, she told an American Family Therapy conference in Miami. "I kept asking myself, 'How can I be here? I've done all these things before in my life. I'm supposed to be settled. I'm supposed to be preparing to be a grandparent.' "

If she'd grown up with some model other than male-biased stage theory, Mason might have been more comfortable arriving at midlife. Instead, she felt odd and out of sync.

This midlife experience of out-of-syncness happens because we are physically and emotionally able to do things that previous generations of women in their fifties couldn't do—or wouldn't.

"A few years ago, just as I was approaching fifty, I took a new job. I moved to a new house. And I adopted a child from Chile."

In the hotel ballroom in Boston, you could hear a pin drop as Carol Anderson, a psychologist and professor at Western Psychiatric Institute, told other therapists what it was like to become a midlife mother. "You have to be prepared to deal with the whole issue of aging and what it means, 'cause kids don't let loose on these issues."

After her new daughter entered first grade, Anderson was preparing to visit Maria's school for the first time and noticed that the child was anxious. Was she nervous because she looked different from her mother? Anderson asked her. Maria gave her mother a level glance and said, "Mom, the kids might say that you're old."

"I said, 'Well yeah, that's right, Maria, they might say that.' "

The girl thought for a minute and said, "Well, I'll just tell them that you're very kind."

Not only are women in their fifties adopting children today, they're actually giving birth to them. On Christmas Day in 1993, a 59-year-old British woman became the world's oldest known mother of newborn twins. Two days later, in Italy, a woman of 63 announced that she too would soon be giving birth.

In Britain, doctors and politicians eschewed childbirth by the postmenopausal and decried the use of fertility treatments for them. These women are too old, they said. "Women do not have the right to have a child, the child has a right to a suitable home," proclaimed the British secretary of health. It is a position espoused by many American doctors who consider women at menopause too old to be able to "guarantee" their children a permanent good home.

"By the thousands," wrote Margaret Carlson in a *Time* essay published shortly after the British uproar, "men over 45 exercise their perpetual rights to fatherhood, marrying and remarrying, having first and second families, without challenge to their right to do so. When it is a man having the baby, few question whether the stress will be too much for the old geezer."

Nevertheless, women who are older when their children are born, studies show, are likely to find mothering more demanding than younger women do. For one thing, they don't have as much social support. Their peers are off on other trails. A 48-year-old mother of a toddler told me it was hard to relate to the younger mothers in the playground. They didn't have the same understanding of life that she did, she sensed. She felt different—*older*—exiled on a park bench by the sandbox with a bunch of women who did nothing but compare formulas. Like Marilyn Mason, this woman was exercising her new midlife options at the cost of feeling painfully out of sync.

But the experience of *discontinuity,* as some call it, is important psychologically, because it allows us to practice change. "Discontinuity allows me to say, 'All right, if I take a new job in a new city, I know how to make a fresh start,'" Mary Catherine Bateson, author of the inspiring book *Composing a Life,* told those attending an Omega

Institute conference on aging held in Manhattan in 1992, " 'I know how to make friends. I know how to reach out. If, heaven forbid, my husband decides he wants to retire in Florida, I can cope with that.' "

Concerns about what's "right" for our age can interfere with and even prevent us from pursuing activities that would broaden and enrich us. Bateson told the women at the conference that resisting pressure from others against doing things *they* consider inappropriate is imperative. Poignantly she recalled how a midlife yearning of her own had been squashed by the ageism of colleagues. "When I was dean of the faculty at Amherst College, they had a wonderful skating rink. I said to some friends of mine on the faculty, 'Gee I haven't skated since I was a kid. I want to learn to do that again.' And you know what they said? 'I don't think it would be a good idea for you to let the faculty see you learning to skate.' "

Consider the very different experience of April Martin, who decided to take her first skating lesson at the age of forty. A "slightly chubby" psychologist and mother of two, Martin says she was only looking for a little exercise when she got bitten by the skating bug. That was five years ago. "Every new step—the first back crossover, the first little waltz jump—was an occasion for such excitement that I didn't sleep for days." Today, writes Martin, "I turn off my alarm at 4:15 every day and stumble to the bathroom planning the two-hour workout to come: I will work on spins and correct that tendency to lean forward on my jump landings."

At 5:20, she is on the ice—an "adult skater," the somewhat derisive term for people who began skating as adults. "We move more slowly, our jumps are lower, our limbs less extended and there is often a touch of fear on our faces." Double-rotation jumps are rare among adult skaters. Triples are out of the question. But adult skaters are athletes, Martin points out. They devote tremendous time and energy to the pursuit of excellence. And they are even beginning to be tolerated by the United States Figure Skating Association.

Martin is fascinated by the contradiction of having "deepened and matured as a woman" in a sport that professionally has been oriented to girls. But though she brings to the ice "the painful bunions and chronically stiff muscles of middle age, I also bring one of its benefits: the increased capacity for living with contradictions.

"My coach bellows across the ice, 'You call that *speed*? My dead grandmother can move faster than that!' "

Martin bends deeper, pushes harder, feels the sweat start to run.

As I read Martin's description in the "Hers" column of *The New York Times,* I got a little chill. On the heels of midlife success and making my first real money when I was 45, I thought I would take up my ice skating where I had left off, at sixteen. Thrilled, I plunked down three hundred dollars for my first excellent pair of custom-fitted skates—Canadian, Reidell boots with CCM blades. I went to Sky Rink in mid-Manhattan and took a lesson. I rotted. I bucked up and took another lesson. I still rotted. I couldn't stand the frustration of wobbling slowly around that large rink, convinced I'd never again be able to do a waltz jump because I was too old. No one told me to the contrary—except my daughters, always supportive, always loving, but what did they know about middle age?

Reading of April Martin's experience made me feel I had given up too soon.

JUDITH Rodin, a researcher, writer, and college administrator, is someone who has reaped great rewards because she was able to transcend age-consciousness, doing things when and where *she* wanted to do them. "I never consciously said to myself, 'I want to get my career established first,' " she says, "but that must have been a large part of why I didn't marry until after I got tenure."

She was 34 when she got tenure and 35 when she married. "I must have been saving myself for myself," she muses.

Single again at 48, Rodin bought herself a house. Not only was she feeling wonderfully self-sufficient, she was dating again. "One of the things I like about [this age] is that I'm no longer trying to be what the man wants me to be, the way we did when we were kids. Now I'm implicitly saying, 'This is who I am—and it would be great if we liked each other.' "

After getting her Ph.D., Rodin had the sinking feeling that she knew exactly how the rest of her life was going to be. She chose not to be bound to a linear, academic path, a decision made possible by the fact that at midlife she had the kind of latitude for development that earlier generations of women, at her age, didn't have. "Here I am in my late forties with a full array of options. I may remarry; I may remain single. I may stay in administration; I may go back to the lab. I may change careers fundamentally, retire early, and do an entirely different kind of writing."

Rodin's willingness to steer her own course has prompted her to make bold decisions. For example, she turned down an invitation to become president of Radcliffe. Why? Radcliffe wasn't what she had in mind. "I realized that if I were to become a university president, I wanted to be president of a large, research-based university," she says. "Radcliffe, with its very unusual relationship to Harvard, isn't really that."

Rodin decided just to stay at Yale and see how things developed. Her self-determination found its reward. In 1991, she was named dean of Yale's Graduate School, and a year later she became provost, making her the highest-ranking woman in the Ivy League.

In that same year, Rodin's book on eating disorders, *Body Traps,* was published. And her name was on the short list of those being considered for the presidency of Yale. During that period, Rodin went on the Oprah Winfrey show to talk about *Body Traps.* Some at Yale criticized her for this, claiming *Oprah* was too lowbrow for a Yale professor. "That's the most ridiculous thing I ever heard," Rodin told *Working Woman* magazine. "Anorexia is a serious disease—it kills women. And *Oprah* reaches a large audience. The idea of calculating everything I do or say because Yale is looking for a president is unthinkable to me."

Yale ended up passing on Rodin, but that didn't halt her rise to fame in academe. In 1993, the year she turned fifty, her alma mater, the University of Pennsylvania, asked her to become its new president. Today she is the first woman to head an Ivy League institution—in spite of, or perhaps because of, having chosen to let her career decisions be guided by her own lights.

Judith Rodin is a radiant example of the adult development model espoused by contemporary psychologists such as Robert Jay

Lifton, who thinks it's better to be resilient and on the move than to be rigid and fixed, however "settled." Nothing is lost by marrying late, divorcing early, and going on *Oprah* to talk about your academic research. At fifty, we have the power to make up our own rules.

TAKING UP WHERE THE GIRL LEFT OFF

IN adolescence, girls enter the age in which they become objects, viewed by society as sexually desirable—*or not*. Thought of as useful and interesting to the opposite sex—*or not*. After puberty, the basis of their social value begins to shift as, ineluctably, they enter the mating game. In the process, they lose their ability to be honest with themselves.

In *Meeting at the Crossroads: Women's Psychology and Girls' Development,* Carol Gilligan and Lyn Mikel Brown write of their fascinating study of one hundred girls at the Laurel School for Girls, in Cleveland. Before reaching their teens, the girls were bright, original, and outspoken, the authors found; but in adolescence something radical happened: A new fear of risk and of disturbing the peace "modified," perhaps forever, their earlier girlish courage, honesty, and willingness to face conflict. Noted the authors ruefully, the teenagers lost "their ability to distinguish what is true from what is said to be true, what feels loving from what is said to be love, what feels real from what is said to be reality."

Honesty, for most girls, is too risky. But it doesn't start out that way. Adolescence—and sexuality—ring the changes, and we spend the rest of our lives trying to regain the boldness we had as girls. It is at midlife, no longer valued for our sexual appeal, that women can regain their youthful courage. "Once past 50," Carolyn Heilbrun writes, "if they can avoid the temptations of the eternal youth purveyors, the sellers of unnatural thinness and cosmetic surgery, they may be able to tap into the feisty girls they once were. And if, at adolescence, the importance of their own convictions had been reinforced, they might, at 50, be ready to take on risk, display a newfound vitality and bid goodbye to conventional limitations."

*   *   *

HEILBRUN'S comment brings to mind Dr. Victoria Elizabeth Foe, developmental biologist extraordinaire. At 48 a recent recipient of a MacArthur award, Dr. Foe looks and dresses, as befits a modern genius, Red Hot Mama style: long peasant skirt and peasant blouse, cowboy boots in which she stands six feet tall, a wild array of black wavy hair. "She has a very unusual character and she has had a strong impact," observes a colleague, "but her style is fundamentally different from the way most science is done today."

A research scientist at the University of Washington, Foe is something of an anomaly in the scientific world. She has never sought a professorship, not wanting the administrative duties. She has never worked for a corporation, not wanting to be bossed. She has neither students nor technicians working in her lab. Her salary comes from the National Institutes of Health, and at the university she does very much what she wants. What she wants is to spend her time peering through a microscope. "There's a deliciousness and a delight to looking at embryos," she told Natalie Angier, the *Times* reporter. "It's a celebratory act, an act of enormous pleasure."

Foe spends half her time drawing what she sees. "Her finely delineated and brilliantly colored diagrams of fruit fly embryos are so exacting and sensual it's a pity they are confined to scientific journals," says her mate, Garret Odell, also a biologist. He and Foe are involved in a major project to detail embryonic growth.

Imagine, as a model for women at midlife, this tall western woman of delicate but strong features who says of her work, "It's like a diver going down into the sea. You notice something new and totally amazing every single time."

If we choose to transcend the limiting shackles ageism would impose on us, personal power, at this stage of life, is something from which we need no longer hold back.

CHAPTER III

CAUGHT IN THE MIDDLE

Where Have All the Children Gone? •
The Midlife Crunch: Juggling the Generations •
Mothers and Daughters in Later Life •
Pulled in Two: A Daughter's Crisis • An Independent Woman •
"He Didn't Want to Deal With the Emotional Part of It" •
An Alzheimer's Story • A Parent Dies (and the Ego Surrenders)

"A THIRTY-EIGHT-YEAR-OLD maintenance man who is into Krishna has been hanging out in my daughter's apartment while she's at work," Catherine told us. "He lets himself in on the pretense of making repairs and stays to light incense. He leaves, of course, before she returns."

On several occasions the maintenance man has called her daughter at night. "I appreciate your fixing the towel rack," she told him once, "but I wasn't happy about the incense." "Oh no?" he said. "And I'd been thinking of staying to fix you dinner."

The next day, Catherine's daughter went to a locksmith, who told her Massachusetts law requires written consent from one's landlord before a lock can be changed. This presented a problem, inasmuch as the maintenance man who likes to light incense is the landlord's brother. Catherine's daughter called her to consult. They decided that as a first step, she should approach the landlord with a simple request for a new lock, leaving out the part about Krishna.

The landlord was said to be out of town for an undetermined

period of time. Catherine's daughter began pushing the refrigerator against her front door before going to bed at night. Catherine called around to see if any of us had valerian.

MIDLIFE begins after the children have been "launched," social scientists tell us. This launching is a pivotal point in many parents' lives. After it (or during it) a great deal may change, especially for the woman whose identity was more bound up with being a mother than with anything else. She may experience what was once dubbed the "empty nest" syndrome, a complex emotional response to children leaving home. Some feminists would like to do away with the "empty nest" concept altogether, considering it gender-biased. That is, it was women who supposedly experienced it; men didn't. Men, enjoying their bigger, richer lives, with so much of import to occupy them, were thought less likely to disintegrate just because the kids were leaving. But after women, too, began getting bigger, richer lives, studies found that they, too, experienced Life After Childcare positively. Studies in the 1970s and 1980s supported "neither the dire rhetoric of the 'empty-nest syndrome' nor the findings of early investigations portraying the empty nest as a time of individual, marital and family crisis," according to sociologist Clifton Barber.

Today, the "empty nest" syndrome is being minimized to the point of nonexistence by academics and television-sitcom writers. Once researchers discovered that not all women come apart at the seams when their children grow up, women's grief over the midlife loss of children was described as a pseudophenomenon. Today, women are supposed to be totally thrilled when their children depart, leaving Mom and Dad free for midday sex on the dining-room table and the blissful contemplation of their burgeoning bank accounts.

But in our effort to view women's lives in midlife as blissful, we run the risk of glossing over the rough spots, where support and understanding would be more helpful.

And women themselves, I learned in talking to them, run the risk of plugging into their children's needs once again, putting their own lives on the back burner. As Willa says, "Just because they're grown doesn't mean we stop feeling responsible for them."

Where Have All the Children Gone?

Catherine says it is something no one but a mother could possibly comprehend: the almost-unendurable tension of not knowing how bad off one's daughter might be while one is on another continent. Catherine had arrived in Venice, where she would vacation by herself for the first time in twenty years. The buildings along the Grand Canal were lit like a backdrop. Watching the ancient city glide silently by at night must be one of life's great experiences, she thought, but fantasies of her daughter's apartment kept intruding: its darkness, its airlessness, the creepy maintenance man.

The problem was that before Catherine left, her daughter hadn't answered her calls for several days. Catherine could envision it, the TV droning, the days-old kitty litter, the answering machine recording an occasional message, but the phone never being picked up. This whole stream of images heightened the phantasmagorical quality of Catherine's trip down the canal in the back of a water taxi, the cabin separating her from the driver, the back of the boat open to the sky, and the possibility of a romantic encounter with the man sitting next to her, whom she had met on the train from Milan. She would like to give in to a new experience, but could she give up the worry? And would giving up the worry mean giving up her daughter?

The man was expansive, European in style, with his arm flung across the back of her seat, his chin tilted up so that he might look at the night sky. A foreign correspondent in Italy for a London newspaper, he was an American who had gained a surface sophistication from his years abroad. He was young, she thought—too young, certainly, for her. And yet, during their hours of conversation in first class, he had made it clear he was attracted. Who, then, riding effortlessly past this glorious stage set, could resist?

But as if some small pleasure might take her, even momentarily, away from her daughter, Catherine was pulled back, reminded of the frivolity of her wish to let it all go, to be a woman mindless—mindless of age, of circumstance, of responsibility, rendered as innocent of consequence as when she was a girl. Yet as a girl she could never have imagined this meeting she would soon have, shutters thrown open to the lapping water, a string of boats below, the seductive mystery, at night, of the Grand Canal, which tells you to go right ahead with whatever it is that moves you. If she were ever going to lose her self-consciousness, her sense of being fifty, her fear of contracting AIDS, this was the moment to do it.

In her hotel, the concierge asked to see the man's passport. Then he handed Catherine a telephone message from her daughter. "I think I need to talk to someone," it said.

It was ten P.M. in the States, Catherine calculated. Maybe they could meet tomorrow, she told her new friend, and went upstairs alone to dial her daughter's number, hoping she wouldn't reach the answering machine once again.

SOMETHING does happen when the nest empties out. Many women told me they miss the chaotic fullness of the years when they were young mothers. And they resent that in mourning the flight of their young birds, they are ridiculed as sad sacks whose lives revolve foolishly and totally around their children.

Even parents who are delighted that their kids are finally on their own will tell you that postlaunch can be a confusing time. Recalling a disturbing visit from her 23-year-old son, Fiona said, "He got off the bus from New York carrying a chihuahua! He talked about it as if it were a baby. He said he had to get right home because it needed to be fed. He was totally regressed. I wanted to lock him in a room and say, 'Don't move. I'll take care of you. I'll take care of the dog. I'm sorry for everything.'"

Patricia, a New York painter and mother of three whose youngest left home only recently, told me she feels the loss of the stimulation her children provided. She hadn't realized how much she'd come to rely on them for the excitement in her life, especially as they got older. Now she has to find other sources of nourishment, she realizes.

Parents in the "empty nest" phase may struggle with feelings of both sorrow and happiness, of mild depression and a fierce wish to hold on. The conflict can produce what sociologists call a "matura-tional crisis," which includes mourning for the relationship that must be let go.

"I liked the arguments," Patricia recalls, "the shouts and tears, those bald intellectual assertions they'd make a dozen times a day when they were teenagers." It's something women thrive on for a good part of their lives—the beehive hum of the kitchen, the blaring stereo and kids dropping in, the smack of the badminton birdie on the back lawn. For Patricia, life had been as rooted in the kitchen shouts and incessant whirring of the coffee grinder as it had been in her painting studio, where she had only the noise of crows for company: "Then I knew that the long stretches of quiet would be bounded by times of intense connectedness with others. Now, there are mostly just stretches of quiet."

Getting the kids launched does, of course, have its rewards. We may feel a freedom we never had before. Our energy can go elsewhere, be channeled into creativity and changed or expanded careers. Marriages tend to improve. Parents are free to be man and woman again. Many experience a resurgence of the passion they had earlier. This is due not only to the lovely new peace around the house, says Clifton Barber, but to profound changes in the couple themselves. Mom and Dad have finally grown up, and—wonder of wonders!—maturity can make love better.

Still, sadness over separating from children is a very real part of the psychological experience of midlife women. We *aren't* as central to them as we once were, and the inner shift we must make is profound. When, after twenty years of being closely tied to our kids, they leave us, remaining connected only by fax, telephone, and the occasional visit, we are affected deeply. Negotiating this loss is an important task. If we back off from the challenge, we can remain stuck in postmotherhood, unable to fly. Many women told me they would feel a pull to become psychologically enmeshed with their children just at that point when they themselves were considering jumping off into something new, something risky, something that scared them.

Could this be one reason so many young adult children today are being welcomed back home to live?

Interestingly, the ones most likely to end up on our doorsteps again are our sons. In 1970, almost ten percent of males between 25 and 34 lived with their parents. By 1980, the figure was 15 percent. The daughters who come home to roost number about half that—and for good reason, according to Brown sociologist Frances

Goldscheider. "The nest is a lot better feathered for boys than for girls."

Adult sons are granted more freedom than adult daughters, she says. In addition, mothers are inclined to give their sons "a totally free ride" on bed, board, and household chores. *The New York Times* talked to mothers around the country whose adult sons lived with them and found that most of the sons felt quite entitled to their princely privileges. "Everything's always done—the laundry, the food—and I don't have to worry about the cable getting shut off, or the telephone," one 27-year-old explained.

God knows it was better than being on his own. "Where I used to live there might be beer cans and pizza boxes stacked up for weeks. And now I drive a Corvette, not a rusted-out Ford Escort."

Good old Mom.

This is the first time in American history that young adults are less well off than their parents—a "fundamental violation of the American dream," as one demographer put it. Some kids come home when their marriages fail. Some live at home because it allows them to buy muscle cars and high-end sound systems—while paying little or no rent.

Mothers who've never worked outside the home are those most likely to end up servicing their adult children, studies show. Fathers, for their part, resent the competition. "All they have to say is, 'Mom, I need a six-pack, twenty dollars, and the keys to the car,' and she's off and running," complained a San Francisco garbageman with 25- and 28-year-old unemployed sons living at home. It infuriated him to return from his night shift and find his giant sons flung out on the couch watching Arsenio. If they can't find an eighteen-dollar-an-hour job, too bad, he says. "They should wash dishes and deliver newspapers."

As people are living longer and having fewer children, "launching" actually ends up being the longest phase in the family life cycle. According to Monica McGoldrick, a well-known clinician and researcher in family therapy, getting the kids launched can last twenty years! By the time they're really functioning independently, Mom and Dad have turned white—or are in their graves.

Today's twentysomethings are often up against major challenges: trying to find cash for the down payment on a house, facing a discouraging job market, perhaps dealing with drug and alcohol problems. Just coming up with the rent for an apartment—which, in big cities, is about what suburban parents face for mortgage payments on an eight-room house—is no easy matter. "It never ends" is a refrain heard frequently from midlife women.

But ambiguity often underlies such statements. Some divorced mothers consider the return of the prodigal son an unexpected dividend. A Houston employment counselor not only gets two hundred dollars a month from her 25-year-old son, she also manages "to get some yard work and car repair out of him." For his part, he is pleased by his new role as man of the house. "I run off her boyfriends on occasion," he says, proudly.

For some women, the so-called financial necessity of having John and Geraldine tucked away in their old bedrooms upstairs can provide a neat rationalization for not taking the risks involved in moving on in their own lives. "People talked to me about 'psychological separation' from my now-grown children," writes Barbara Grizzuti Harrison, who after her divorce lived with her children for twenty years in an eight-room apartment in the Park Slope area of Brooklyn. "I was stubborn: Italians don't separate, I said, until they get married—then they move down the street."

But Harrison knew things were getting too tight as she scrutinized her adult kids' comings and goings, "peered into their faces as they watched TV," and listened to them as they turned in their beds at night. "We practiced the little, corruptive deceptions, the sincere pretenses of people who love one another profoundly but live too close."

The time had come, she decided, for someone to make a move. "Go for it, Ma," her son said, and she took it as a blessing and moved out. Now she lives in a small apartment in Manhattan from which she can see the Empire State Building, and she loves living unobserved. Not that things exactly stopped dead with her children. When her daughter talked about possibly moving to California, Harrison asked, "Are you running away from me?"

"Not everything is about you, Ma," the young woman replied.

THE MIDLIFE CRUNCH: JUGGLING THE GENERATIONS

IT isn't unusual for women approaching fifty today to have the launching of their children still ahead of them. In fact, they may only recently have *had* their children. Thus, when their parents begin to fail, these women experience responsibilities that threaten to dominate their lives. It doesn't make any difference what economic class you're in, how educated you are, or how caught up in a profession: Midlife today exerts a double whammy.

Ours has been called "the sandwich generation." In a study of women whose median age was a few months under fifty, gerontologist Elaine Brody found that four-fifths were married, while the remaining 20 percent were widowed, separated, or divorced. *At fifty, 84 percent of the women still had one or more children living at home, and 20 percent had a parent living with them.* Three-fifths of the women in the study were working, and over half were providing some degree of caretaking for their mothers.

A much larger government study found that 30 to 40 percent of those in their fifties with children were helping them, and a third were helping their parents financially or in other ways. Contrary to popular myth, elderly people in this country are not shunted aside. Rather, they remain in very close contact with their children. In one study, 85 percent of elderly parents saw or spoke to their children two to seven times a week.

The children that parents talk to, however, are most frequently daughters. Sixty percent of adult daughters play the role of confidante, helping sustain their elderly mothers emotionally. But then, adult daughters are confidantes and caretakers to everyone in the family, notes Monica McGoldrick in *Women in Families.* "They take care of their husbands, their children, their parents, their husband's parents, and any other sick or dependent family members."

Day in, day out.

Job or no job.

Single or married.

*   *   *

The gritty ones do it with humor. Angel, a 51-year-old grandmother who lives with her female partner of eighteen years, has recently discovered that with increasingly dependent aging parents, children and grandchildren, and health problems of her own, she has a lot on her plate. Angel is the head honcho in her family, it has recently dawned on her.

A late-night emergency brought it all home. "My grandson had swallowed a coin. Of course my daughter called me. I'd been in the city all day and was exhausted. 'Come to the hospital,' my daughter said, and I ran to the hospital at ten o'clock at night. They were all there—my son-in-law, his two brothers, my younger daughter, everybody. I looked around and I realized that the doctor was addressing himself to me with whatever he had to say. I went, 'Oh my God, what do I do here?' So I ran down the hall and spent ten bucks in the junk machine and bought candy for everyone. I thought, 'Well, that's about the best I can do.' "

Everyone ate the stale candy, the baby cheerfully survived, and in the midst of the chaos, Angel had one of those midlife epiphanies. "I realized I was the matriarch of this group, and that I would be on call like this for the rest of my life."

The "dependency squeeze," as McGoldrick terms it, only gets tighter as the years pass. Not only are children financially and emotionally dependent on their parents far longer than they used to be, but the parents of today's midlifers are living longer. A friend from college whom I hadn't seen in a while told me her mother is in her nineties now and living in Florida with her two sisters, also in their nineties. "They're living together, I assume," I said.

"Oh no," my friend replied. "Each has her own condo. They'd probably kill one another if they lived together."

Mothers and Daughters in Later Life

When my mother was 85, I flew south to take her to the beach for a few days. Six-year-old Nicky, whom I consider my grandson (his mother and my son live together), accompanied me.

We stayed five days in a house on the edge of a marsh. At first, I thought it might have been a mistake to force the generations under one roof. ("You don't think he might be a bit hyperactive?" my mother asked after our first hour together.) But in a day or two, it seemed the most natural thing in the world for two women, aged 85 and 55, and a boy of six to be eating together, talking in the early mornings, and going up the stairs to bed at night. My mother and I would take Nicky swimming in the morning and again in the afternoon. I would take him bike riding in the long evenings. "Why doesn't Gladys ride with us?" Nicky asked. "She used to ride a bike," I explained, "but now it's too hard for her."

One night a band came to play by the ocean. They were a young black group from the low country south of Charleston, and they danced like MC Hammer. Parents and children of all ages convened by the ocean to listen. The group played its keyboards and steel drums in the moonlight. The kids danced as if they'd been dancing since the day they were born. My mother sat on a plastic beach chair, a bright scarf tied gypsy-fashion around her head to keep her hair from blowing in the wind. I perched next to her, with Nicky on my lap. It was a magical experience.

The next day my mother said, "It's odd. I just haven't realized how depressing it is to spend all your time with old people." This was not self-pitying but a statement of fact. The old are segregated. "I wish there were something we could do about your being in the retirement community," I said. "Well," she replied, "it's just the way it is."

As it turned out, she didn't want to leave Sandpiper Village; this was where her friends were, she said. Not long after Nicky and I returned north, my mother wrote that the community had gotten a new activities director who promised "intergenerational activities." "I think that means we get to spend time with children," she said, dryly.

The amount of competence that some very old women retain is astounding. My aunt, at 92, was still taking care of her invalid husband at home. She did the wash, the cooking, and the housekeeping and tried to keep him cheered. When it came time to grocery-shop, she hopped into her electrified golf cart and went for it.

My mother enjoys helping some of the others in her retirement community, walking a blind friend around the compound for exercise, driving groups to the harbor to see the ships. But with a blood condition that eventually will be fatal, her own health is cause for constant concern. I find myself becoming angered by the close-mouthed doctor who tells her little about her plummeting platelet count, and wonder if she'd be better off in the care of someone else. Yet I know such decisions are hers to make. She says she wants to stay with this doctor, she's used to him. I tread a narrow line and call her a lot.

WITH over two-fifths of older people living at the top of a four-generation lineup, today's women-in-the-middle are likely to be the second or third generation in a family. Those in generation two have responsibilities to the very old, as well as to children and grandchildren. Women in generation three have responsibilities to their children and to *two* generations of older people, their parents and their grandparents, and/or their in-laws.

The drama of the demographic change stems not only from the increased proportion of the older population—from 4 percent, or 3 million, in 1900, to 11 percent, or 125 million, at present—but from the way the older generation is aging. Their lives are not only longer but more complicated. The times they are a changin'—for them, as well as for us.

Joanne and Willa's mother, Florence, age 72, called Joanne from Florida at seven o'clock one morning to announce that she was having "a romance." Someone in her complex—"a Spanish man," she said—was meeting her at five o'clock every morning for a walk. Today, she said, they held hands for the first time.

There was a pause. "Does Daddy know?" said Joanne. "Yes," said her mother. "Daddy doesn't care."

As soon as she hung up, Joanne called Willa, waking her up to tell her that their mother was taking walks with a strange man in New Century Village at five o'clock in the morning. "What I want to know is," said Willa, "are we ever going to get free of this?"

*   *   *

By the time they themselves reach the age social scientists refer to as "young-old," adult daughters find they are taking on more and more responsibility for aging parents. The parent who'll likely need them longest is Mom. By the time they reach 75, women outnumber men in the population by almost two to one. In her final years, an old-old mother becomes increasingly dependent on her young-old daughter. Mom will do what she can for herself, but her daughter may do much of the rest: paying the bills, organizing food, dealing with laundry, cleaning, and doctors, shopping for mother's underwear. As the two women age, the daughter's caretaking tasks become more extensive. Women in their forties help their aging parents an average of three hours a week. By the time they're in their fifties, the figure is up to fifteen hours a week. When they're in their sixties, the still young-old daughters are providing, on average, twenty-three hours of parent care a week. These are not facts that we usually take into account, or even talk about, in planning our postfifty lives. No one expects Mother, or Mother's sister or mother-in-law, to swerve suddenly into our lives, all stops pulled, needing financial, emotional, and practical help with the most basic details of living. But suddenly, there it is. . . .

PULLED IN TWO: A DAUGHTER'S CRISIS

LOUISE had worked for two decades when she decided to quit her job and start a family. Why not? she said. She'd paid her dues. She'd waited all her life for this baby, the white house and the picket fence, and now she was going to have it all, full time, no compromises. "You can't have it all at once," the new saying goes, "but you *can* have it all serially."

Maybe.

Louise had spent her twenties, and then somehow her thirties, going from one job to another, trying to find a way to support herself and at the same time express her artistic talents. She did a brief stint in her husband's retail store (part of her brief stint in a first marriage). She worked as a rug designer, dressmaker, cocktail waitress, and jewelry designer's rep, and she assisted a famous New Age guru in his home office. But beneath the job-hopping lay a single dream: a husband, a family, and the luxury of staying home and watching her baby grow.

No sooner did Louise enter her second marriage, at 39, than she began trying to have a child. It proved a difficult process. As soon as she became pregnant, she miscarried. Two more miscarriages followed. Louise began thinking seriously about quitting work. "It was crazy to be schlepping heavy jewelry sample bags when I was trying to get pregnant and bleeding."

It was also not part of the dream.

Louise and Jared began the long process of trying to accomplish artificial insemination. "I must have been inseminated with his sperm a dozen times," she recalled. The clock had just about run down. Then a friend offered to be a surrogate mother for them. How could Louise possibly refuse?

The rationales for accepting the offer were right there, ready and waiting. It would be stupid for her to pursue another career, Louise told herself, when what she really wanted was to stay home and be a mother. And there was so much to be done around the house—they couldn't really afford to hire someone else to do it. "Jared was totally behind me. He said, 'Just stop that job. You're not making much money. Forget it, stay home and take care of me.' I said, 'Great!' "

Louise was 45 when Juliet was born from the surrogate mother. She had already begun menopause, but no matter, she had her dream—a hard-working husband, a child, life as a stay-at-home mother. Jared, a dentist, initially supported her wish to be a full-time wife and mother, but as the 1990s rolled in, money got tight and he began to talk about how much better it would be if she went back to work.

But working with a baby in tow hadn't been part of the dream. And besides, this was a woman who had her hands full. Several months after Juliet was born, Louise's recently widowed mother came to live with them. Suddenly there it was: Louise was plop in the middle of the sandwich generation and swaying with hormonal changes to boot. "I had two babies to take care of," she says. And then, thoughtfully, "Really, three."

Jared is a traditional husband, a workaholic, out three nights a week or more. "Professional meetings," says Louise, "things he really has to go to if he's going to make contacts." He also travels on weekends. "He has to do some of this," she explains, "but I think he's taken it to extremes. The bottom line is, he's not around that much."

Louise, 48 now, is so busy she scarcely has time to notice whether Jared's around or not. Juliet, not yet three, is too young for nursery school. Louise's mother is eighty. "She was kind of frantic about living alone for the first time in her life. Even though she managed the family finances before my father died and was the driving force in the family, she didn't do well without my dad. So she came and lived with us for a while."

After a few months Louise's mother entered a fancy retirement community, where, she found, social life was structured into unfriendly cliques. Although she could afford the rent, she felt outclassed by the other residents, who, dressed to kill, treated all meals as if they were major social events. It got so that she hated entering the dining room, where she'd have to look around to find a table to sit at. As the weeks went by, she began staying in her apartment rather than sit at tables with chattering strangers. More and more she depended for her social life on her daughter.

Louise was sympathetic. "I would include her as much as I could in my activities and my errand running. In the morning I'd call her up and say, 'Well, this is what I'm doing today. Is there anything you'd like to join in on?' Or 'Is there something you need that I can get for you?' 'Well,' she might say, 'I'd really like some new bras.' So I'd fill that into my schedule for the day and take her shopping for underwear or whatever. And she could come up with things, believe me."

Louise's brother wasn't greatly involved when it came to caring for his widowed mother. As she analyzes her brother's inadequacies, Louise rationalizes the unfair burden placed on her and perhaps feels a bit superior: "I don't think he ever separated from my mother, and so he can't deal with her on a person-to-person basis. I did my separating years ago so I can take it with a grain of salt. Even though she's a pain, I still love her because she's my mother."

For two and a half years Louise saw her mother every day. "At times I thought, 'What have I gotten myself into here?' I felt stretched by two babies with extremely different needs. I was constantly between the two of them, trying to keep them apart in a way." Mom resented the attention Juliet got, and her babyish demands. "She really expected Juliet to be much more grown up than she was," says Louise. "They were battling for my attention whenever they were together, and I was doing my best to satisfy them both."

Where, in this stressful mélange, was Jared? "Poor Jared was just left out in the cold a good deal of the time. I was too exhausted to deal with him, and he's a very demanding person who was used to getting a lot of my attention." She was glad her husband was seeing a therapist, Louise says. "At least he gets some attention there."

The pity for her husband that Louise expresses masks anger at his lack of involvement. She herself was wiped out. "Emotionally I felt drained, as if there were nothing in my own life that was for me. It was all about my mother and Juliet and Jared."

To get solace, she returned to the teachings of Da Avabhasa, a spiritual path she'd followed years earlier during periods of crisis. "It allowed me to feel that I had a little life of my own somewhere."

But she got to have this life only after she crashed at night: She'd read a little from her guru's teachings, then fall asleep. "He gives you guidance in every area," she explains.

Louise hangs on to a glimmer of hope about the future. "I do have an idea of what I want to do when I have a little bit more time," she says. "I want to start designing painted folding screens for the design trades."

Her new dream sounds more like a self-consoling fantasy than anything that will really change her life. If she had it all to do over again, would full-time motherhood really be her dream come true?

"Well, the reality of it doesn't fit any of my pictures," she says, laughing ruefully. "Of course, I didn't anticipate having my mother with me when this little dream took place."

And then, in a rush, it all tumbles out. "I don't think I would recommend this to someone else. It's too late, I really think, to have children. It takes all my energy just to keep it going, keep Juliet going, the house going, take care of Jared. Well, certainly to take care of my mother. It's worn me out."

Louise feels as if she's getting old fast. "I don't know if I can recapture my energy before it's too late." Worse, she has begun feeling like a house martyr. "I'm married to this house, you know." She expects great things of herself, but all the demands on her seem to obliterate her ability to concentrate. In that respect she's like all mothers of young children. It doesn't matter that she's close to fifty.

"I used to be organized, but forget it, I can't do that anymore. I can't find things. My house is a total jumble. I'm managing on a day-to-day basis. I can keep it all together—in a very diffuse way. The balls are still in the air, but barely."

On balance, Louise thinks she might have said to herself after the miscarriages, "Nature is telling me something here. Like maybe you're not supposed to have kids when you're this old."

An Independent Woman

STILL, while the new demands of midlife are challenging, they can bring gifts, surprises, nuances of relationships with loved ones that you never imagined possible.

My mother had been in the hospital twice, that winter, with a bladder infection that sent her temperature soaring to 105. The second time around, her doctor finally got the clue that antibiotics weren't working. He called in a urologist who measured the intake and output of her liquids, ascertained that she wasn't voiding completely, and recommended regular catheterization.

When the time came for my mother to learn how to catheterize herself so that she could leave the hospital and go home, Jan was the nurse she picked to teach her. Jan claimed to have had twenty boyfriends since she left her husband, and to know how to drive an eighteen-wheeler. Jan is 56 and a free spirit. My mother liked her style. They were a kind of Thelma and Louise of Assisted Living. Without Jan, my mother might never have been able to locate her urethra. With Jan, it became an adventure in self-knowledge, poignant not least because it was happening to a woman born just after the century had turned.

"God, Mom," I said, impressed. "You've never even used a dia-phragm, have you?"

"Diaphragm?" she rejoined. "I've never used a tampon!"

Now, at 86, she would be catheterizing herself twice a day. The doctor had told her she was "savvy" enough to do this, and she found it empowering. "The main thing," she told me after her initial lesson, "is keeping the field sterile."

"Don't worry, Ma," I said. "Keeping things sterile was always your specialty." She had been big on attacking germs for as long as I could remember.

When I got my mother home from the hospital, doing a catheter-ization was the first order of business. I wasn't sure what role I was to play when she came out of the bedroom, and asked me for help. On the carpet in her room she had set up her "sterile field": a disposable pad provided by the medical supply company, balls of cotton, and betadine, which squirted projectiley from little individual pouches when you tried to open them. The catheter was a red rubber tube about a foot and a half long, the tip of which gets inserted into the urethra while the other lies in an open plastic dish. It's a straightfor-ward enough procedure, providing you can find the entrance to the urethra.

First came the thing we both feared most, the frank look at the perineum. My mother was lying on her back on the floor, craning her neck to try to see in a hand mirror what was what. She'd been taught to begin by swabbing herself with cotton balls dipped in betadine. "Down the center, front to back," she intoned, "then one down the left side, one down the right." A handy diagram showed the urethra lying midway between the clitoris and the vagina. But it was nowhere near as visible to the naked eye as the diagram made it appear. We pressed into action the emergency road lantern my brother had given my mother for Christmas.

On her first try, she missed. In her position on the floor, she wasn't able to see much of anything. I sat on the edge of her bed, my hands folded in my lap, trying to be supportive but not intrusive. After several more unsuccessful tries, she asked me to get down on the floor next to her and see if I could find it. My heart went out to her as she lay there with the skin on her hips and stomach stained with streaks of the wayward betadine, but she seemed bent only on mastering the procedure.

I got down on the floor and peered. The task of finding the urethra was made more challenging by the fact that my mother's uterus was prolapsed—a portion of it appeared like a shiny red egg at the entrance to her vagina. With the lantern shining on the egg, it looked, I told her, like the diamond displayed in Tiffany's window. She laughed. I placed the tip of the catheter against the spot that looked vaguely right and gave the barest little shove. Suddenly, miraculously, urine began to flow. It emerged from the end of the rubber tube and began pooling in the plastic pan. *"Yes!"* I shouted triumphantly, fist in air. My mother smiled.

That night, after getting ready for bed, she came out to the living room and thanked me for everything. "Think nothing of it," I said. "I consider it a bonding experience."

"I think this goes beyond bonding," she said.

You might think that by the time a woman reaches eighty, the urogenital tract would be less of an issue. Not so, not so at all. "All the ladies drink cranberry juice," my mother said of her compatriots at Sandpiper Village. Word had reached this outpost that cranberry juice helps prevent bladder infections. "At dinner, you can look around the dining room and see all the red glasses."

"Oh God," said Willa, when I told her. "Is this what we have to look forward to, sitting around with the Mamas in our eighties, drinking cranberry juice?"

Willa's apprehension is what we all feel as we watch our mothers go through the final trying stages. "There but for the grace of God"— and the grace is only going to last so long. I try to understand this part of my mother's life. I try to have a feel for it, sadnesses and all, and not back off out of anxiety about my own mortality.

"The doctor says I may have to have surgery," my mother says, "but I don't know. They say the results only last for a while."

"A while is what we're talking about here," I say.

"That's true," she says. "As the doctor said to the woman, 'You don't expect to live forever, do you?' "

IT'S long been acknowledged that mother-daughter relationships are critical to the well-being of older mothers, but the reverse, it turns out, is also true. In a 1991 study published by the Wellesley College Center for Research on Women, Rosalind Barnett found that the greatest wish of some adult daughters is that their parents might finally come to know and understand them as they have always yearned to be known and understood. The women Barnett studied expressed a desire for support, acceptance, and love from their parents more frequently than they expressed a desire for respect and mutual affection.

The daughters Barnett studied were part of a random sample of a larger study of employed women living in eastern Massachusetts. Most of them lived close to their parents: 63 percent lived less than half an hour's drive away, and 15 percent lived within one block. Contact between the generations was frequent; over half the parents saw their daughters every week, and 12 percent saw them every day. There was also plenty of telephoning. Eighty percent of the parents spoke to their daughters weekly or daily. "Not surprisingly," says Barnett, "fully 73 percent of the parents said they were very satisfied with the frequency with which they saw their daughters."

Interestingly, while the daughters thought what they were getting from the relationship was equal to what their parents were getting, the parents thought *they* were getting more than their daughters.

"HE DIDN'T WANT TO DEAL WITH THE EMOTIONAL PART OF IT"

THE culture we live in doesn't acknowledge the many pressures with which midlife women simultaneously contend. Two-fifths of adult children, most of whom are daughters caring for an older person at home, *devote time equivalent to a full-time job.* "To an extent unprecedented in history," observes Elaine Brody, "roles as paid workers and as caregiving daughters and daughters-in-law to dependent older people have been added to [women's] traditional roles as wives, homemakers, mothers, and grandmothers."

The convergence of two major social phenomena—the vastly increased number of older people in the population and the growing proportion of middle-aged women in the labor force—has placed midlife women in an unprecedented situation. A huge study released in 1993 by the National Institute on Aging found that on average, daughters do two and a half times the caretaking of parents that sons do. And many do a great deal more. From early adulthood, says Monica McGoldrick, women are taught "to stand by their men, to support and nurture children, and paradoxically, to be able to live without affirmation and support themselves."

Sons may offer financial help, supervise property, and help with funeral arrangements, but daughters provide the day-to-day care, even though most of them work full time. "They shop and run errands; give personal care; do household maintenance tasks; mobilize, coordinate and monitor services from other sources, and fill in when an arranged care program breaks down," reports Brody.

These data shouldn't be construed as signifying that sons lack "responsibility or family feeling," Brody states rather questionably, but instead that they reflect "the cultural assignment of gender-appropriate roles."

It is interacting with others that keeps empathy alive. Whether or not they're "assigned" the roles they play, men who remain detached from the needs of other family members inevitably end up with their feelings less engaged. A vicious cycle ensues. The less engaged they are, the less they "see" that other family members need their help. Unfortunately, "the way it is" gets validated as the way it's supposed to be.

At 48, single, with a son in engineering school, Marla has a hairdressing salon in a small town in upstate New York. "Marla is a caretaker," says a friend, and *caretaker* being one of those all-purpose twelve-step words, it isn't immediately clear whether her friend admires Marla for it or holds her in disdain. Marla's, in any event, is the story of a woman who puts others first. It is also the story of a woman who never got, and could never quite push herself to ask for, a fair shake. At midlife she seems to be playing out the role she has always played—that of the giver who doesn't get.

As a girl, Marla showed signs of being artistically gifted. In high school, she thought she would like to study art in college and become an advertising designer. But she had five brothers. "If anyone was going to go to school," she says, "they would go first."

Marla never got to school. Once she married, her husband had to be put through college. That's when Marla began cutting hair. "It seemed better than both of us struggling to work and go to school at the same time."

Marla supported her husband through four years of college, after which he got a government job in Washington. By then, they wanted a family. Unable to conceive, they eventually adopted a two-week-old boy and Marla stopped working. "My husband said he'd be making enough money. Of course I wasn't thinking of divorce. I wasn't thinking I'd end up raising this kid all by myself. And that the struggle of putting my husband through four years of school was not going to benefit me later."

The marriage ground to a halt when Marla's husband decided he didn't want the baby anymore. Jimmy had developed asthma and become difficult to care for. "The emotional stress was just too much, and he wanted me to give the baby back," Marla recounts. "It was almost like, 'I proved I love you by letting you have the baby. Now you prove you love me by giving the baby back.' I didn't think that was a fun game to play."

Going back to school was now out of the question; Marla was on her own with the baby. The man at the salon where she worked convinced her that, with a very sick child, she should "cultivate the gift I had with hair instead of trying to reach out for something else." Marla fought for child support but got nothing of their joint assets for herself. "I didn't fight for it. I should have fought, but I just didn't. I signed the papers and gave him what he wanted and just walked away."

So hairdressing it was. Marla continued with it until Jimmy was twelve, when she decided it was time to move him up north to be closer to her family. Marla's ex, after maintaining a sporadic relationship with Jimmy over the years, no longer wanted to see him. It was because he'd gotten angry at her, Marla says, for seeking through the courts—and being awarded—financial help for a therapeutic summer camp for the boy. "A doctor told me that when your father doesn't want to see you, it's like he doesn't love you, and you're no good. So we moved up here, where Jimmy could get a sense of love from his grandparents." Marla hoped her son would never figure out that his father didn't want to see him.

Once upstate, Marla opened a small hair salon in the back of her house and kept on trucking. It turned out to be a wise move. Not long after they left Washington and the off-again-on-again scene with her ex, Jimmy's asthma disappeared. In six years, he was ready to enter one of the toughest engineering schools in the country. After he left home, Marla had her place to herself for the first time in her life—though this didn't last long. No sooner had she accomplished the herculean task of rearing her son than, like clockwork, both her parents began to fail. "My mother has liver cancer and a heart condition," she says. "My father has congenital heart failure, arthritis, and poor vision. He's eighty-nine. Both of them have trouble hearing."

Her father didn't drive anymore, so food and medication had to be gotten for the elderly couple, and their animals needed care. At first, Marla and one of her brothers did the helping. "We made a pact that we'd put our lives aside for a while in order to take care of them," she says. Then things became more and more demanding, and Marla thought it would actually be easier if she just moved in with them for a while.

Almost immediately after she made this decision, her brother decided to split for California. "What about our pact?" Marla asked. "I put my life aside for long enough," he replied. "There's nothing on my birth certificate says I'm an only child, and I gotta get on with my life."

Marla's brother had little empathy for *her* desire to get on with life. "You get your rent free," he said. "What are you worrying about?" That attitude really shocked Marla because her brother had always been so crazy about his mother. But like Louise, she took comfort in rationalizations. "I think he really doesn't want to be around to see them die."

Still, she also sees the injustice. "I thought to myself that it was just like with my husband and son. As soon as Jimmy got sick, it was a whole different thing. My husband wanted out. He didn't want to deal with the emotional part of it."

So Marla, once again, is dealing with all the parts, emotional and otherwise. And for it, she gets little appreciation. Her father resents her help and criticizes her for not doing things the way he used to do them himself. He complains that she doesn't use the washer and dryer properly. "They think I'm just a girl and I don't know how to do anything. I say, 'I'm a mature adult woman. I have washed my clothes. I've washed my husband's clothes. I've washed my son's clothes. I have been on my own for years now.'"

This argument is lost on her father, who has only one fear: If the washer breaks down, there won't be money for another. So Marla's mother uses the washer for their clothes, while Marla, accommodating to the end, goes to the laundromat to do hers. Worse, her father has gotten it into his head that Marla is sponging. "When I come home from work, he leans over to my mother and stage-whispers, 'Let 'er fix her own dinner,' " she says.

What she finds most stressful of all is the antagonism between her parents and Jimmy. "There's so much tension between them, he wouldn't come home from school this vacation," she says. Nothing the poor kid does is right, as far as his grandfather is concerned. He doesn't push in his chair when he leaves the table. He doesn't put things back in the refrigerator in the same place he got them from. Marla's almost-sightless father wants to know that his pitcher is on the first shelf, far right, where it always is. He can't bear having his routine disturbed and grumbles constantly at his grandson.

Marla tries to assert herself. "I said, 'Look, this is my joy. My son is my joy. I've come here to help you, but I just can't let you take away the only joy I have by creating friction while he's home.'"

Marla wants to be in her own place again, to find out, for the first time, what it is like to be on one's own, not dependent on anyone. Jimmy, she recognizes, has been something of a crutch. "You know, when a man comes over, I say, 'Well, you have to leave now because my son's coming home.' I don't know. Maybe I moved in here with my parents because of that. But I'll never know if these things were crutches or whether this was actually what I wanted unless I try going it alone."

At the same time, the family situation makes it difficult for eighteen-year-old Jimmy to accomplish his task of psychological separation. When grandparents are still alive and functioning but failing in health, the family anxiety level can become very high. What goes on between the parents and grandparents may stimulate confusion and resentment in the young, which makes their task of separating more difficult. None of this is lost on Mom.

A friend of Marla's told her her parents had just lived too long. It was a disturbing notion. "No," Marla insisted. "I mean, you don't want to see your parents gone. Yet you think, 'Yeah, she's right, maybe they *have* lived too long at this point.' What do you do? You want to go on with your life."

That's key: You want to go on with your life. Women at this age can become discouraged when their personal agendas are disrupted by the caretaking needs of others. Because women often don't demand that men share in family responsibilities, they end up in what one report has called "enmeshments of ineffectiveness" with their children, or parents, or siblings. Overwhelmed by all the demands, midlife women can get caught in a web where their unsuccessful attempts to be everything to everyone affect their self-esteem.

But who is to blame here, the women for not fighting, or society for not helping them? Is Marla's "enmeshment"—with her demanding parents, her nonempathic brother, and her son old enough to leave home but still too young to provide her with any external support—an example of "ineffectiveness" or of overload?

An Alzheimer's Story

As Monica McGoldrick points out, the laws regulating social services that might support families are written mostly by men. These laws don't support women, who bear the burden of family responsibilities yet wield no power. The failure of the government to provide public services to aging families, McGoldrick thinks, is exacerbating the intergenerational conflicts that lead to elder abuse.

Too much is too much, in other words. Some women—like the daughter who abandoned her Alzheimer's-ridden father in a wheelchair outside a racetrack rest room with a box of Pampers in his lap—snap.

OF all the women I interviewed for this book, those whose lives were the most difficult were coping with parents with advanced illness and Alzheimer's. In such families, everything that has once seemed relatively simple becomes an overwhelming chore.

"When I took my mother into Philadelphia to visit the doctor, she was horrible," said a woman I'll call Evelyn. She and her husband, Robert, live outside the city on the Main Line. Evelyn's mother, who is living with them, has turned irritable, hostile, and unpredictable. She has been in that state for months, and things are getting worse. "Her paranoia is driving us mad," Evelyn says. "She calls us thieves. She was going to take me to court. She said she wanted to tell everyone in town what I was doing to her. There are times when all this has a real nightmarish quality."

It's one thing to grasp intellectually that one's mother has become a different person, Evelyn will tell you; it's quite another to remain emotionally calm in the face of it. You never know what's going to come next. "In a split second there are these incredible mood swings. Recently my mother said to me—Robert swears he heard her say—'You fucking bitch.' And then she came into the kitchen and heard me as I was telling my brother on the telephone about the retirement community I'd looked at for her. She started yelling, 'Go to hell, go to hell!' I snapped. I said, 'I *am* in hell, I've got you!' She can't hear me. Thank goodness she can't hear me."

But Evelyn's mother didn't have to hear. The next thing Evelyn knew, she was hitting her mother: "I punched her arm. She didn't feel it as much as I did. It was a nightmare. I couldn't believe that I could do that. I mean, I've *thought* about doing it any number of times, but never did I think I had the capability of actually doing it."

Evelyn and Robert are hoping to improve their situation by creating a private space for her mother in their house. "She's very reluctant to be moved. See, she's upstairs on the same floor with us now, and we want some privacy. So we're fixing up the space downstairs. It's really one of the nicest places. It's the brightest and warmest in the house. And it's perfect. And there will come a time when she's not going to be able to negotiate steps anyway. So why change her when she becomes disoriented?"

But she's resisting. "To her, it's kind of like being cast out of heaven into purgatory. But for us, it's our salvation."

Evelyn's mother has begun going through her daughter's personal things and scrutinizing the mail every day. "She thinks we're stealing her mail. She reads my mail all the time. Nothing is private. Now I'm telling Robert, 'Let's put padlocks on the doors so she can't go into our spaces and invade them like that.'"

Evelyn's friends, who know that she's had a poor relationship with her mother since childhood, wonder why she doesn't just put her in a nursing home. "One of them said to me, 'Oh, you're just going through this selflessness, this martyrdom, keeping your mother with you.' I said, 'Well, I don't look at it that way. I'm not viewing it as martyrdom.' There's a part of me that wants to get rid of her, that would like to dump her. But that's not the biggest part of me. The biggest part of me says, 'This is my mother. She's a human being. I want her to have her dignity, what's left of her dignity.'"

Regardless of the way her mother has always treated her, says Evelyn, "she's still my mother. I'm her blood. I came from this woman. I am a part of her. She's a part of me. To deny that is like denying myself. I can't do that. I don't really think I could do that to anybody. I've worked in nursing homes. I've seen what they're like. They're not all the same, that's true, but my mother is a very difficult person. I know that with her personality, she would easily be singled out to be abused because she's so abusive and so cruel herself—she'd be a primary target. So in a way, I'm just protecting her, doing the best I can to protect her. I know that this is how I would want to be treated."

Yet Evelyn has a terrible fear of buckling under the strain she's experiencing. "I want to make sure that I don't become one of those people who degrades and dehumanizes another person, because I *could* do it. I'm sure I have that potential. Because you can be driven to it in the end. I'm surprised by what I'm capable of doing, and yet I'm not surprised at all. But I know that I won't hit her again," Evelyn insists. "Because I didn't hit her. I hit myself. That's who I hit. That's who I hurt." She begins to cry.

Evelyn has finally joined an Alzheimer's support group, but even there she feels alone. "I'm the only one in my group who's chosen to have their loved one live with them. Most people just don't want to do it. And I can understand it. I cry when I give her a meal. I sit and watch her eat and see how tiny she's becoming. I look at her face, and I see she has a small face. And I'm seeing her in a way that I, unfortunately, never saw her before and will never see her again."

Most people in the Alzheimer's support group say the hardest part is "when they don't recognize you anymore." But Evelyn says, "To me that won't be the hardest part. This is the hardest part. Watching her go, little by little, piece by piece."

A PARENT DIES (AND THE EGO SURRENDERS)

WHEN we are younger, we imagine that the death of our parents will be devastating. This is true no matter how difficult our relationship with them may be, and it reflects our own insecurity more than any devotion we may feel. We see ourselves as weak and vulnerable, and we imagine that when a parent dies, a part of us will die, too. And we wonder whether we'll be able to survive.

Though I had feared it since I was a small child, my father's dying became, unexpectedly, a kind of gift. Not his dying so much as what happened between us in the weeks leading up to it.

THAT he was a difficult man, no one would contest. He was brilliant, arrogant, bristling with defenses. For years he did scientific research while teaching at a university. Growing up, I sensed that he was interested in me, but I was never really sure about his love. Men like my father don't communicate their emotions. His letters, when he wrote at all, were maddeningly general. On the telephone, it was *his* ideas he wanted to talk about, not mine. For a long time I took this to mean that my ideas were not important enough, my concerns and tasks as a woman beneath notice. I have spent my life trying to understand why he would think this, why Father always came first.

Marion Woodman, a Jungian psychologist and writer in her seventies, compares such a parent to King Lear. "I'm sure some of you must know this kind of father or mother," she said at the Omega Institute Conference, "Conscious Aging." "They come to your home to visit, and they expect to change it into *their* home. What do you do?" Woodman asked. "How do you handle such a situation?" For her, that is the central question of Shakespeare's *King Lear:* How does an adult daughter give up her power struggle with her father, without losing herself?

The Lear-fathers themselves suffer, of course. Like many men of his generation, my father had found the core of his existence in work. But once he retired, he was left with few resources. "Lear has been king. He has ruled by power," said Woodman. "Who are we when we have to give that up, and how do we move from a position of power to love?"

As the years passed, my father became increasingly abstracted, and by the time he reached eighty, he seemed quite despondent, although he still feigned cheerfulness. He tried to write, but the spiral notebooks we found in his bedside table showed the paucity of his thought in the last months of his life, his inability, simply, to expand on anything. Such intellectual constriction is a function not of age, we now know, but of illness. Often, for older persons, that illness is depression.

A year before the accident in which, somehow, he managed to pull away from a stop sign into the path of an oncoming truck, I had taken my parents and children to the beach for a few days. My father had always loved the ocean, but this time he refused to put on his bathing suit. He wouldn't even come onto the sand but remained under the pavilion, dressed in his seersucker suit, his panama hat, and the black shoes of a style he had worn for fifty years. He sat in a beach chair holding a drink he barely touched, staring out past us, past the ocean, past, even, the horizon; in a sense, he wasn't there.

But when the accident happened, he fought. He actually got out of his car with five broken ribs and walked to the ambulance. He called my mother from the hospital and told her not to worry. Then his lung collapsed.

Eighteen days on a respirator is a long time, and the nurses in intensive care wondered from the beginning whether he'd make it. At the end of the day he would have what seemed like panic attacks. The doctors thought they might be related to the pain-killers. He suffered, as well, from intermittent visions, angels on the ceiling, children in the corners. Once, when the doctor and I were standing side by side at the foot of his bed, he thought the doctor was my husband, long dead. He wanted to know whose baby that was between us. I had to say, "Dad, there is no baby." I had to say, "Dad, it's not Ed, it's the doctor."

Children and babies seemed very much the stuff of his thoughts. One evening when I was visiting him alone, he asked if he could have a baby with me. I told him I was too old to have children. "You are?" he said. "You look young to me." I thought that he might have thought I was my mother. I thought that he might have known quite well I was his daughter. It didn't matter. He was old, he was on morphine, and who knew what was going on in his mind, in his hopes, in his soon-to-be-long-lost dreams.

After fifty years of fighting my father, his powerful influence, his grandiosity, his disturbing shifts in mood and need for attention, I wanted now to give him everything. I went to him during every visiting period, telling him again and again that I loved him, telling him how wonderful he was, how important to me. Because of the respirator he was unable to speak, but he responded by squeezing my hand and using his face to communicate amusement, irony, doubt. I would hold a notepad for him while he painstakingly printed questions. Where was my husband? Who were those children hovering toward the ceiling? Was he ever going to get well?

We relate to others through our suffering, Woodman says. We make the move from power into love through the opening caused by a breaking heart. Suffering ends the "judge-and-blame games," she says. "You recognize your own humanity. You recognize the humanity of those around you."

As the days passed, my mother, my brother, and I grew exhausted with the strain of worrying about my father, but I was as unmindful of my physical state as if I were falling in love. I would fly north to take care of my work and fly south again a week later. My father was off the respirator but still struggling. Late one night, driving home from the airport, I was aflame, as if the car were a chamber permitting me a feeling of calm, intense focus. Earlier, as I was taking my leave, my father had turned to my mother and said, "There goes the laughter and the sunshine." As I drove home on the Thruway, that statement of his returned to exalt me. My father and I were on the same wavelength! We were communicating as we had never communicated when he was well. There was nothing between us now, no anger, nor disappointment, nor even yearning—and I knew as clearly as I have ever known anything that this was a gift.

The heart breaks, says Marion Woodman, but in the breaking it opens to love.

ONE day in the nursing home, where he had been sent to recuperate and to learn to swallow again after his long agony on the respirator, my father began to vomit. The nursing home didn't call the doctor, though my mother asked them to. My father vomited for a day and a night before an ambulance was finally sent for. Only after he was back in intensive care was it discovered that his feeding tube had become disengaged. The plug that had held it in place had fallen back inside his stomach, and his esophagus had been blocked for twenty-four hours. The pneumonia he contracted because of having aspirated vomitus was far worse than the pneumonia he'd gotten after his lung collapsed.

When he'd been back on the respirator and in a coma for ten days we had a meeting with the doctor and head nurse and said we wanted my father taken off the respirator. They agreed. They would leave a T-bar of oxygen in front of his mouth, in the unlikely event that he was able to breathe on his own.

My mother decided to go home while this happened. My brother and I stayed with him. We each held a hand and listened to my father's FM radio. When the announcer said that the piece about to be played was Strauss's "Homecoming," we just looked at one another.

There had been no squeezing back for days, and while I held on to my father's still-warm hand, I knew that in a way he had already gone. My face was wet with tears I didn't feel myself cry. I was looking out the window, past the heavy machinery being used to build a new addition to the hospital, and into the horizon. For an hour, we watched the monitor as his heart rate slowly but steadily dropped. The nurse, a man, came into the room and stayed with us, watching, until the final zero appeared on the screen. Then, with maddening efficiency, he began unhooking everything. Couldn't he wait? I wondered; but then it seemed pointless to wait.

My father died on Valentine's Day. It was a miracle to me that my heart had opened, that finally I could think of him without bitterness or regret, could love him without stint.

MIDLIFE is a time to let go of old grievances. Marion Woodman told us that years ago, in England, her psychoanalyst once said to her, "You know, Mrs. Woodman, you're going to go down that path whether you like it or not. You can go like a squealing pig towards the slaughter, or you can go consciously and with as much grace as you can muster."

"The point," said Mrs. Woodman to the midlife women—Lear's daughters all—sitting before her, "is that the ego surrenders, opens the heart, and in that opening new energy comes in."

CHAPTER IV

"THIS IS WHAT FIFTY LOOKS LIKE"

APPEARANCE, LIVELIHOOD, AND SEXUAL SELF-CONFIDENCE

The Betrayal of the Body • Who Is That Stranger in the Mirror? •
The Politics of Appearance • The Big Lie: Passing for Younger •
Negative Images • The "Dangerous" Age •
Pathologizing Midlife Desire • I Dream of Chin Hairs

EVERY THREE MONTHS or so, I slip into a building on lower Fifth Avenue to visit Mary Ellen Brademas, a dermatologist who is treating me with a medication that—mirabile dictu!—tightens pores and diminishes wrinkles. I feel as if, in the interests of preventing the solar keratoses to which I am prone, I have stumbled upon the goddess.

"Work on them, work on them!" Brademas advises. Like a cheer-leader urging the team on to greater effort, she encourages more religious application of Retin-A to the lines on my upper lip. Her own example is hard to ignore. A smooth-skinned and beautiful blonde in her fifties, a mother of three who went to medical school at age 38, Brademas is associated with New York Hospital. Fancy Fifth Avenue office be damned, she gets *down* with her women patients. "My upper lip looks weird when it's peeling," I say. "Oh, I'm constantly peeling myself," she says, airily waving off my complaint.

Brademas told me on my first visit that she pumices herself in the shower every day, "from the tip of my toes to the tip of my chin." She seems to view the aging body the way she views everything else: You're in charge of it, it's not in charge of you.

Getting into the swing of things, I admitted my concern about the little skin tags that seemed to be multiplying on my back. I didn't like the possibilities. By the time my father reached his seventies, the same rubbery little blobs had covered his back like some hardened layer of antediluvian rock.

"Don't worry, there's medication for that," said Brademas efficiently, proffering a prescription for lotion. "It's kind of like a body peel. It does for your body what Retin-A does for your face."

I cast off my robe and started dressing. "You're in great shape, Dowling," she said appraisingly, arms folded across her chest. "How old are you?"

"Fifty-five." A part of me felt proud, but I also felt self-conscious, wondering how long "great shape" would be accurate, or if, indeed, it was even accurate now.

"I'm older than you," Brademas announced cheerfully.

"Don't rub it in."

"Oh, I'm not rubbing it in." She believes that looking young is a matter of how hard one is willing to work for it. I believe it's a matter of genes, and Brademas's are obviously better than mine. My mother, in her bathing suit, looked like a calendar girl into her seventies. My father turned white and skin-tagged before he reached fifty. I take after my father.

The Betrayal of the Body

Susan had put on weight. She kept thinking she could drop it if only she could get back to the gym. She was living in a kind of time warp. Something was out of kilter. When she looked in the mirror, she felt no congruence with the image she saw. The short choppy haircuts she used to get away with seemed too butch now, so she was growing her hair long. Something in her wanted to insist she could get herself looking the way she had twenty years ago, a tall jeans-wearer with auburn hair swinging straight to the waist. Now, with her hair at this in-between stage, she ended up mostly tucking it behind her ears. Thick bangs grazed her eyebrows, dragging her face down. Her whole image was out of whack. People still took her for younger, but she'd given up on style as her facial features loosened. She didn't care, she would tell herself, as she pulled on her Birkenstocks in the morning.

She did care. "The over-forty beauties in *People* say they do it with exercise," she told Willa. "They swim, jog, bicycle, and dance aerobically. Ali MacGraw says, 'It's like brushing my teeth. If I don't do it, I go crazy.'"

"There are things driving me crazy, too," Willa said, "but not that."

In honor of her fiftieth, Willa had joined a dating service. She'd described herself, on the application form, as "a pleasing combination of muscle and curve."

Susan felt she had muscle and curve all right, but the combination was no longer pleasing. When she went to the gym, she'd work out like a demon, but while she'd tone up a bit, she could never quite drop the weight. Discouraged, she'd kick back for a month or two, then start keeping the gym bag at the ready, waiting for the inspiration to address her sagging gluteus once again. Her husband Scott said he didn't mind her butt, but she minded. She really minded. It looked as big as the side of a barn in almost every sweat top she owned.

Susan was a high-level hospital administrator and had felt successful, actually powerful, for years. But now she lacked *presence*. She was feeling uprooted, anxious about what was happening to her, confused about what the future would bring. The hourglass had tipped, and her self-esteem was on the wane. On the wane, hell—it was crashing. A woman who had spent her youth being looked at, Susan was aware that people—men, especially—had stopped checking her out as she walked by. In fact, they didn't even seem to be *seeing* her. Was the reason Scott didn't give a damn about her butt that *he* wasn't really seeing her, either?

* * *

A woman arrives at midlife to find that the eye of the viewer has become doubly demanding. Now, besides being pretty, she is expected to look "young." It isn't age so much as the appearance of age that matters. "We define someone as old because he or she *looks* old," says historian Lois Banner, of the University of Southern California, in her study of women, aging, and power, *In Full Flower*.

In the days—and this was only decades ago—when women were jeered for losing that ephemeral beauty on which they had staked everything, the coming of maturity was like a death knell. What worth, they thought, could they possibly have at fifty, even forty? No one needed them. No one thought them attractive. No one even noticed them walking by on the street. Men, as they matured, grew bellies and chins and had oil portraits painted of themselves. Women covered themselves, hid their bodies, bewigged their thinning hair, and painted their faces with bright blue lids and off-center jolts of lipstick—all in the effort not to be written off.

No wonder the sight of our bodies beginning to age brings horror. Older, for a woman, has traditionally meant worthless. It has traditionally meant sexless, and even faceless. We were brought up on these views, and thus, even though times presumably are changing, we still try to keep ourselves looking young. Or if not young, at least healthy, at least high-energy and thin. Entering one's prime may have become hip, but *looking* as if one has entered one's prime is as anathema as ever.

A woman can find something frightening about her changing appearance. She worries about losing the glisten, the shine, the soft blemishlessness that gave her her feeling of purchase on the world. She loathes losing the high round curves, the well-placed muscle, the veinless white skin. She mourns the loss of her thick lustrous hair, that halo that had always made her *come out*, have presence, be, in a sense, bigger than she was.

On top of all the physical changes, she worries that she's neurotic. Normal, well-adjusted women simply slap on the estrogen cream and forget about it. Normal, well-adjusted women don't obsess about the deepening fold between nose and chin, the stomach that bulges, the veins that splotch the inner thigh. Normal women accept aging the way they accepted menstruation, the fatigue of the ninth month, the tender postpartum episiotomy, the cracked nipple, the diaphragms and gels and tampons, and mopping themselves up in endless Thruway rest rooms. *Normal* women, a psychiatrist would tell us, *like* getting older, or at least they accept it, seeing the lost uterus, the nonfunctioning ovaries, and the wrinkled turkey necks as trade-offs for the joys and mysteries of maturity. But can that psychiatrist produce one woman—today, next week, or next year—who in fact has made this "adjustment" painlessly? I don't think so.

WHO IS THAT STRANGER IN THE MIRROR?

"I was sitting in a session one day with a new patient, and we were working on some transference," Emma, a psychotherapist, told me. "I asked him something, and he said, 'Well, what I see before me is an attractive middle-aged woman.' That really hit me. I mean, this man is in his early thirties, and he sees me as an attractive middle-aged woman. I froze in my seat. He was right. I *am* a middle-aged woman, an *attractive* middle-aged woman, but *middle-aged.* 'Oh my God,' I thought, 'that's me!' "

It was one of those little epiphanies that begin hitting us relent-lessly at midlife. Things have changed: I am not being viewed in the same way. *Men* are not viewing me in the same way. This—whatever this is—is the new me.

To be a woman no longer young is to be twice over "the other," Simone de Beauvoir wrote in *The Second Sex*. She meant that aging women are doubly objectified, once for being female and once again for aging. The more we have relied for self-esteem on compliments about our looks—and society sets us up for this—the more likely our confidence will erode as youth and beauty fade.

Blanche DuBois, in *A Streetcar Named Desire,* may have been an extreme example of the older woman devastated by the loss of the only value she thought she had—her sexual appeal. But the poignancy of her character stemmed from the universality of her plight—at least in the 1950s, when Tennessee Williams wrote the play. In the 1990s, a woman like Blanche would be considered extremely ill. Yet how far are we today from the anxiety she experienced as an aging woman? To keep ourselves sane, we still have to fight media images of aging women who, thanks to makeup and filtered lights, offer the illusion of rip-roaring youth.

When we were young, Twiggy was the ideal of femininity. At midlife we have Lauren Hutton, who's in her fifties but looks 35 (at least in fashion photographs). Being told incessantly that she's really over fifty only makes the rest of us fretful. It's not unlike what happened after Gloria Steinem told a reporter who remarked how young she looked, "This is what fifty looks like." That comment, touted in the press, became an anthem to the youthfulness of the new midlife woman. Suddenly, although this certainly was not Steinem's intention, women had a new and impossible ideal with which to compare themselves. Who could blame some of us for sulking silently, "Maybe this is what fifty looks like for *you*, Gloria . . ."

The point is, fifty doesn't look like anything. Or shouldn't. The idea that a certain way of looking is "normal" for a certain decade—or even, heaven forfend, a certain specific year!—has got to go.

THE double standard hits hardest at midlife. "Men are not really any more interested in you or your life than when you were young and cute—not unless you're Margaret Mead or Sandra Day O'Connor," says Vietnam reporter Jurate Kazickas, who, at fifty, has not exactly had a dull past. (An episode of *China Beach* was based on a true story about Kazickas getting blasted with shrapnel during the war.) "At dinner parties they do not look at you and think, 'Well, she's old, but I'll bet she's led this really interesting life.'"

The effect on women's psyches of the sudden loss of attention might be compared with what happens to them physically when they stop producing sex hormones. It's as if a switch were thrown and a changed state entered. What *is* this? What happened to me? Who is that stranger in the mirror?

Some women ultimately give up on getting attention, adopting the "at last I can be myself" position espoused by Gloria Steinem and

Germaine Greer. "Since society casts us aside, we can finally become ourselves after fifty," Steinem said when she was 59.

Others refuse to go out with a whimper, attempting instead to maintain their attractiveness by lifting dumbbells, undergoing plastic surgery, and/or lying about their age.

The degree of disturbance a woman experiences is of course variable, as is the particular "aberration" around which her fears seem to crystallize. Some of us abhor the wrinkles, some the stomach, some the varicose veins. "I had no idea that your lips get smaller," says actress Ellen Burstyn. "I'd never heard or read one word about that. But I kept noticing something different every time I put on my lipstick, and then I realized my lips were shrinking."

Since her face was in part her fortune, Burstyn felt her shrinking lips to be more than an indignity; they represented a potential loss of income.

Midlife body changes that signify masculinization are the most likely to turn women obsessional. "I have two pieces of chin stubble I've been plucking for three years," says Honey, a grandmother in her fifties who has worked as a bookkeeper for thirty years and plans to retire, she says, *never*. "I watch for them daily in my five-times magnifying mirror."

She watches and she wonders. All the advanced moisturizing creams in the world won't prevent midlife chin growth from feeling ominously like beard. Should she "move on" to a wax depilatory? It isn't her husband she's worried about, Honey says; he is tactful at least. It's her grandson, who at five, having a tendency to tell it like it is, is likely to blow her cover, shrieking in some public place, "Yuk. Your face is scratchy!"

And if that happens, Honey says, she is going to feel *old*. Not only old, but worse: mannish.

Gender is the issue with midlife hair growth—as it is with hair *loss*, which can be traumatizing, especially for those who for years have thought of their lush manes as adding to (if not indeed *creating*) their femininity. "See what you can find out about this," a photographers' agent I know whispered desperately, as if she had contracted a rare disease whose cure might be buried in the stacks of the medical library. "I watch my hair go swooshing down the sink drain, and I could cry."

(Women who are farther along on the postmenopause road refer with wan humor to their thinning pubic hair. I know a woman of seventy who attributes her balding pudenda to the vigor of the sex she enjoys with her husband of forty years. Her friends can't bring themselves to suggest that her aging biochemistry is the culprit.)

Many of the physical changes we experience at midlife, from hair loss to dry skin to alterations in weight, are caused by menopausal shifts in hormones. Since these interact with our body chemistry, the sum total of menopause's effects are quite individual. Some women end up with a beefier testosterone presence in relation to their remaining estrogen, for example; while they're more likely to sprout new facial hair, they'll also be likely to retain good levels of libido and energy. (See Chapter VI.) Women who enter menopause with more body fat tend to manufacture more estrogen, postmenopause, than those who are naturally thinner, and as a result they'll be less vulnerable to hot flashes, insomnia, and mood swings. The physiological changes that menopause triggers are so individuated, unpredictable, and—especially in the event of hysterectomy—so sudden that midlife can bring on feelings of vulnerability not unlike those that hormone shifts produced in us at puberty.

The year she stopped having her periods, Electra, a New York actress, watched with fascination as her breasts became small and flaccid, her face rather bony. In the beginning she liked her new angular look. "It reminded me of myself at adolescence, long, lanky, and small-breasted. But after a while I began thinking I looked more like Katharine Hepburn in her declining years—her scrawny body, that is, not her wonderful face."

Electra began taking estrogen supplements, whereupon her new lankiness reversed and she became zaftig again. Beyond zaftig, Rubenesque. "It happened so suddenly, my initial reaction was shock. I was in Washington to do a play, and I stopped into a Victoria's Secret to get some bras. It had only been three months since I'd been bra-shopping, but now my 34B was miserably inadequate. Spongy, dimpled flesh was spilling out on the sides from beneath my armpits. I'd never seen anything like it."

Unique to a woman's body is its vulnerability to swift, hormonally induced weight changes that can result in a precarious sense of being out of control. Puberty, menstruation, pregnancy, postpregnancy, menopause, postmenopause: Throughout adult life there are the swellings and bloatings, the sudden onset of sponginess that recedes just as suddenly once bleeding begins. Being content as a woman requires being able to adjust to these shifts in weight and body composition, to accept rather than be undone by them. But no one ever talks to us about this, and so we receive little validation for the normalcy of the shifts in our appearance from one week to the next. It's possible to spend one's life fighting the body's natural changes.

Soon after Electra began the hormone supplements, a surprise dividend appeared. "My face plumped up just enough to smooth my skin and make the wrinkles less noticeable. I glowed with a kind of pregnancy glow. My agent said, 'I would think you'd had a face-lift, except that I know you haven't had the time.' This was thrilling to say the least. My breasts filled out and regained their 'turgor,' a word I didn't even know existed until I lost mine."

But just as Electra had begun feeling reborn—another menopausal hormone shift! Now suddenly her hips, thighs, and abdomen were looking loose as jelly. One day Electra found herself in a position she'd spent her entire life avoiding. "I was trying on clothes in a tiny cubicle of a dressing room, and my mother was sitting right there with me, facing me at stomach level. I said, yanking the dress over my head as fast as I could, 'I've really put on weight.'

" 'Well, I must say,' she replied, as if on cue, 'I've never seen you looking so . . . *bulbous.*'

"I decided to up my exercise, lower my estrogen, and never again get stuck in a dressing room with my mother."

Women, accustomed to fighting for beauty, tend to redouble their efforts at midlife. "I will *not* be fat at forty," they say, and they mean it.

See these same women at the gym at fifty, and they're thinner than ever. But men, conditioned to believe they remain dashing no matter how many chins they develop, let it all hang out. Health, energy, and erection capability may be issues for them, but not wrinkles. Less likely to equate sexual attractiveness with how young they look, men give up sooner.

But they don't want their women giving up. "I'm attracted to beauty in everything," explains a 240-pound aesthete, a man of fifty who takes it as a sign of his increased maturity that he's begun dating forty-year-olds. He prefers it, however, if they don't *look* forty. He cites the extraordinary physical abilities of his most recent girlfriend, a woman of forty who looks thirty due to the fact that she does every one of her yoga moves while standing on her head.

A divorced 57-year-old who's been having one-night stands all his life told me he's looking for more stability now that he's pushing sixty. Younger women, he admits, are making him feel nervous about his sexual prowess. These days, he prefers to be with someone who has had "the same number of years on the planet." In exchange, he'll put up with a few flaws. "I'm kind of attracted even sensually to gray hairs," he says—"wisps of gray hair."

What about chunks? I ask. He smiles sheepishly. He's not too interested in chunks. *His* hair, of course, is almost totally white.

THE POLITICS OF APPEARANCE

THERE are reasons why this business of looking older is so haunting to women. Women today must work through their sixties and beyond, supporting themselves and members of their family in a society that continues to deem aging women impaired. Yet society's negative view of aging women affects our ability to make a living—our likelihood not only of holding on to a job but of rising in the ranks, being respected and rewarded for the maturity we bring to our work in the same way that men are.

A woman of fifty who is looking for a new job or a promotion "can be undercut if she appears old," says Marilyn Yalom, senior scholar with Stanford University's Institute for Research on Women and Gender. Burdened by graying hair, wrinkles, and expanding waistlines, women can find themselves being treated "like wilted produce." "This emphasis on looks is really a disservice to women because it hurts access to employment and how women perceive themselves," says Joan Kurianski, executive director of the Older Women's League.

A New York courtroom lawyer who has a face-lift scheduled says she's quite clear about the reasons for her decision. "It's not the judges whose response to my aging I'm worried about. They're trained to look past appearances to people's core," she says. "It's the juries I don't trust. I have to go up against male lawyers, for whom age heightens authority in most people's minds, while women who show signs of age are considered out of it. This is a reality. Should I buck it in the interests of some presumed greater integrity? No way."

PARADOXICALLY, to reap the rewards for having matured, midlife women have to *look* as if they haven't matured—or at least haven't matured "too much" (the "too much," as always, determined by the eye of the beholder).

Tom, a management consultant who works with Fortune 500 companies across the country, explained to his wife, writer Marcia Seligson, why it's so important for upper-management women to make themselves look younger. "If you are the age of the mothers of the people you're supervising," he said, "it's hard to have an adult-to-adult, nonmaternal relationship with them." Whose problem is this, one wonders, the midlife woman's, or that of adult employees functioning on the emotional level of children?

Privileged, by virtue of her husband's connections, to hear the way executives talk about the people they hire, Seligson says that for women, "Seasoning, maturity, and experience have less cachet than I would have assumed."

Which is putting it mildly.

In *The Beauty Myth*, Naomi Wolf tells about a 54-year-old woman who lost her job without warning because her boss said he preferred to spend his workday looking at a younger woman "so his spirits would be lifted." The tough news today, says Seligson's management-consultant husband, "is that if a woman wants a management job, it behooves her to look as rested, relaxed, and youthful as she can."

"Translation?" says Seligson. "Face-lift."

Recently I saw a remarkable play, *Two Faced,* in which Lyn Adams, who wrote and performed it, played a middle-aged woman abandoned by her husband. Distraught over the assault to her identity, she couldn't get anyone to hire her. Her daughter convinced her that a "makeover" would change the job market's response.

The audience, sitting beyond the fourth or "mirror" wall of the woman's dressing room, watched as the actress laboriously went through the steps of applying the most amazing battery of "aids" to her aging face and body. After clipping store-bought cheek-lifts to her sagging skin and hiding them beneath a wig, applying makeup and double eyelashes, and putting on a push-up bra, beautiful hosiery and, yes, a girdle! this woman emerged young. Upon seeing the final transformation, the men in the audience gasped, almost as if they'd been let in on the secret for the first time. The females tittered and groaned. And of course the woman got a fine job, pronto, and a new lover.

But in the play, only a relationship with another woman puts the abandoned woman at peace with her gray hair and roundish belly. And gray, smiling, and softly wrinkled was how we found the actress/playwright in the back of the theater, after the performance. I grasped her hand and thanked her for her play, then wandered out into the rainy night feeling that if nothing else, something hidden and dark for us had been publicly acknowledged.

The Big Lie: Passing for Younger

After teaching elementary school for thirty years, 52-year-old Anne, who lives in a small river town in upstate New York, is looking forward to early retirement. Her husband Dave, a periodontist, is about to retire. They've been married twenty-eight years and have two grown children and an eighteen-month-old grandson. When asked how she's experiencing this transition into her fifties, Anne, an attractive blonde who clearly takes pains with her appearance, says, "I'm still fighting hard."

"To?"

"Be thirty-five. But I expect someday I'm going to give up, because I don't have the energy."

Anne fights the aging process by exercising, coloring her hair, controlling her weight, and trying "to keep an open mind." If she had more money, she would "fix her stomach" with plastic surgery, she says, so she wouldn't have to work so hard at holding it in. "I suppose if I were eighty pounds overweight with a huge appetite, I would give up on all that," she says, "but I'm just close enough to stay in control."

It's hard to keep up the fight against fifty when one of your kids ups and makes you a grandmother. "At first I was embarrassed," Anne says. "I didn't want anyone to know I was that old. But the baby is so nice. I'm glad we have him. He calls me Anne. I don't tell him to call me Grandma. When I'm with him, people think he's my kid and I don't tell them otherwise."

"Grandma" is an image that Anne wants no part of. "At work, I've always lied about my age," she says, "automatically taking ten years off when I had to fill out forms. But then, when I had the chance to apply for early retirement, the truth had to come out." At first no one believed her, Anne says proudly.

But she couldn't rest on her laurels. To keep from becoming "nonexistent," she takes courses by the handful. She wants to feel smarter than the other women in her circle. She thinks she needs the edge. Most of those women are married to her husband's friends, and they're second wives, some much younger than she. She worries about standing out, being different. "I don't want them to look on me as if I'm his mother," she says, although actually her husband is a few years older than she. Anne feels at a disadvantage. Older men want younger women and younger women don't mind being with older men; they *like* it, in fact. "They see Dad and security, father with his glasses on."

* * *

Elaine—petite, energetic, dark-haired—has a hard time admitting she's 54. "I don't say it to anybody," she confided soon after we met. Divorced, with two grown children and a high-paying career in computer sales and marketing, she regularly lies about her age, both at work and in her relationships with men. "I hate lying. I don't lie about anything else in my life, and I don't do it like a liar does. I do it to play this game of life in this very strange world where they have these expectations and doors close on you because of your age."

When Elaine meets people, she never knows how old she's going to say she is but decides on the spot the best age for the situation. She got off on this track almost immediately, she says, with a man she met at a party. They started talking at the buffet table and had barely approached the steamer roast when the subject of age came up. Elaine made a quick estimate of how old the guy was and lopped two years off that, telling him she was 45. "That's kind of what they like," she says. "Two years."

Apparently her calculation was on target. The two became an item. Eventually, of course, she had to tell him she was six years older than he. While at first he found the news upsetting, mostly it made little difference, she insists. Quid pro quo. "He admitted to me that if, that night at the party, I'd told him my real age, he might have spent the evening talking to me but he would never have called me."

Their relationship lasted a year, but recognizing that they had no future together, they parted on friendly terms. Several months later Elaine began a new relationship with a lawyer who was 45. At the time I talked with her, he hadn't yet broached the horrifying subject of age, but things were getting tricky. When she introduced the man to her 28-year-old daughter, Nikki, Elaine shaved a year off her daughter's age and said she'd been married at nineteen. So far, he's still in the dark. And she's convinced herself that when she finally has to tell her lover how old she is, it will no longer be an issue. "I don't think he's going to break up with me just because he finds out I'm actually nine years older."

But Nikki up and got married, and now Elaine is contemplating how she's going to deal with it socially when her daughter decides to have a child. "I think I can say I'm a grandmother without revealing how old I am and still be able to fit into the world that I seem to be playing in," she muses.

Let them think that she was very young when she had her daughter. Let them think her daughter was very young when *she* became pregnant. It may be a dysfunctional way to live, but some women prefer it to the insecurity they experience when telling the truth about their age.

The world Elaine is "playing in" is Silicon Valley, with its computer deals, high-tech patents, and driven, self-absorbed youth. Everyone she works with, including her boss, is under forty. When Elaine needs to use her birth date as a computer password, she has trouble remembering it because on her personnel record she lopped four years off her age. Did she lie because she thought it would affect whether she got the job? No, she says. At that point she'd already been hired. "It was more a feeling of wanting people to keep seeing me the way they see me."

How do they see her? "As young and kicky."

STAYING young and kicky in Silicon Valley (or anywhere else, for that matter) can probably put years on you. Women like Elaine are trapped; trying to feel good by "staying young" is a strategy that leads to a dead end. As Betty Friedan points out in *The Fountain of Age,* "The attempt to hold on to, or judge oneself by, youthful parameters blinds us to the new strengths and possibilities emerging in ourselves."

Elaine says she just doesn't want her age to be an *issue.* But it's an issue in her own mind long before it becomes an issue in anyone else's. *And* the clock is ticking. She plans to give her current relationship a year. "Meanwhile, I'll be getting a year older. Then I'm fifty-five and I'm less marketable."

In defense of Elaine and others like her, it requires saying that the ability to maintain self-esteem as we age is very much influenced by the culture's way of viewing women. In the few societies where women experience little or no increased status as they get older—and ours is among them, sociologist Pauline Bart found—sexual attractiveness invariably is valued more highly than craft ability, technical knowledge, or wisdom.

No wonder aging, in America, makes women feel precarious.

Negative Images

Susan Sontag once wrote that there is only one standard of beauty for females, and that is the girl's; but males have two standards of beauty, one for the boy and one for the man. Thus, as men grow older, they are "able to accept themselves under another standard of good looks—heavier, rougher and more thickly built. . . . There is no equivalent of this second standard for women."

Society's images of midlife women are powerful and often negative, and they influence us in ways both subtle and obvious. To counter them, we try to insist triumphantly, "I am *not* my mother at fifty," and while there is some truth to the statement, there is also, within it, a lie. We *are* our mothers at fifty, for the compelling reason that our mothers are our most powerful models—for aging as for everything else. How they felt about themselves as they aged, the options they believed they had, their vigor, energy, and optimism—or lack thereof—inevitably color our own experience.

Not only must we deal with our current social reality, then; embedded in us like an evil charm is society's view of older women at the time when our *mothers* were turning fifty. Part of us fears that even though the look is different, we may be just the way our mothers were at 48, in their windbreakers and slacks, pushing their carts up and down supermarket aisles, still yearning for a life, furious that their time is up. They have no luscious odor or lascivious laugh. Their hair is salt and pepper, drying as it coarsens and thins. As they check the packages for ounces and cents and caloric value, they are all earnest calculation. They have chores to do and households to manage, and they will do these chores and manage these households until they no longer have the strength. God help them.

Why did our mothers, most of them, become so asexual at midlife? Some scholars—among them historian Lois Banner—have suggested that women of the previous generation more or less "de-sexed" themselves at the age when society considered it dangerous, without children to tie them down, for them to continue behaving sexually. "Accordingly," Banner writes, our mothers "became shapeless figures who cut their hair short, wore stout shoes and clung to out-of-date polyester fashions as part of the grandmother role."

To add insult to injury, these de-sexed women became the stuff of caricature. *New Yorker* cartoons featured the "clubwoman"—heavy, shapeless, and infantile at midlife, a creature institutionalized in the 1940s by the cartoonist Helen Hokinson. "In her drawings," writes Banner, "the clubwomen have only a childish understanding of the world, of sexuality, of men, of themselves." That cartoon image, she believes, came from a destructive fear of female aging.

The full fury against the modern midlife woman emerged in 1942, in Philip Wylie's *Generation of Vipers.* "Never before has a great nation of brave and dreaming men absentmindedly created a huge class of idle, middle-aged women," wrote Wylie, who was beside himself in categorizing the "hot flashes, infantilism, weeping, sentimentality, peculiar appetite, and all the ragged reticule of tricks, wooings, wiles, [and] subordined fornications" of menopausal women.

Lambasted by today's feminists, Wylie's popular book was influential in the 1940s. Social scientists—male and female—climbed on its bandwagon, proclaiming midlife women childish and insubstantial. Erik Erikson himself wrote that "remnants of infantility join advanced senility to crowd out the middle range of mature womanhood, which thus becomes self-absorbed and stagnant."

Given the histrionic attitudes that prevailed, it isn't surprising that women were terrified of being "caught" aging and remain so to this day. Recently, when a reporter asked the actress Madeleine Kahn how old she was, she "went into what only could be described as a catatonic stupor," wrote *The New York Times*'s Michael Specter. " 'I hope you wouldn't print information like that,' she said, looking at the floor as she spoke. 'It's not a normal question.' "

Flustered, Kahn babbled on. " 'I suppose you have the right to print the information but I would prefer that you did not. I mean it's not important. And I would just request that I be treated like a lady and not have it specified.' "

Cannily, the reporter offered no reassurances. "The silence got pretty loud after that," says Specter. "Then she burst forth again: 'I mean let's face it. This is still a factor in a woman's career. And it shouldn't be. But it is. I just wish that one didn't have to be diminished by facts like that.' "

At the end of the story, Specter told his readers, "Ms. Kahn is 51." Her presumed vanity in not wanting her age revealed was only heightened by the stunning photograph that accompanied the article.

How silly of this woman, we were supposed to think. Bright, talented, beautiful, and on top of her career—and she's worried about losing it?

It wouldn't be the first time a middle-aged woman was made to seem ridiculous for worrying about her age.

The "Dangerous" Age

In the days when *The New Yorker* started publishing its trivializing cartoons, the clinical view was that menopause could drive women mad. It was "losing the true female function," psychiatrists believed, that popped us over the top. Menopausal women were supposed to be vulnerable to a unique depression that resulted from their inability to conceive anymore. "Consciously and unconsciously," wrote Edwin Hopewell-Ash, "the whole female organization rebels at the abrupt ending of reproduction." Supposedly of a deteriorating nature, this "rebellion" was formulated by Emil Kraeplin in 1909 as a diagnostic category: involutional melancholia. It remained on the books until the American Psychiatric Association's *Diagnostic and Statistical Manual* finally dropped it, in 1987.

In the 1930s, 1940s, and even 1950s, involutional melancholia was said to be rampant. Zelda Popkin reported in 1953, in a scholarly article, "Widows and the Perilous Years," that *most* psychiatric hospital admissions were menopausal women whose diagnosis, invariably, was the purported "involutional psychosis."

Undoubtedly some midlife women *do* suffer psychiatric disturbances, and some require hospitalization. But the view then was that menopause made women *in general* go out of control.

And who, we might ask, was naming the kinds of behavior deemed, for women, irrational? Often it was doctors. "When a woman of 48 shows signs of alcoholic intemperance, a craving for drugs, or becomes 'converted' to a new religious creed, begins to exhibit an indifference to her husband and children, neglects the home, develops a passionate zeal for the emancipation of her sex, or falls ardently in love with a youth . . . these . . . are ascribed to 'the change of life,' " one conservative physician in the 1920s claimed.

My own research indicates that if we substitute a craving for experience for a "craving for drugs," these very "symptoms" would constitute the perfect litany of possibilities yearned for by midlife women today. Yet views like this physician's were so pervasive in the first half of the century, not even an emancipated thinker like Simone de Beauvoir escaped them.

De Beauvoir's particular mentor was the noted Freudian Helene Deutsch, whose ideas about menopausal women infiltrate *The Second Sex*. Seven years earlier, in *Psychology of Women* (undoubtedly the most influential text on the subject at that time), Deutsch had written that menopause triggers in women a return of adolescent, even juvenile behavior. De Beauvoir had a heyday with this idea, sounding at times almost as vitriolic as Wylie. Describing the pathetic (if oppressed) menopausal woman as wishing desperately to "get into action again," de Beauvoir acidly mocked the "second youth" notion ("one and all, they declare they never felt so young") and berated women for dressing young, assuming childish airs, and trying to persuade others that the passage of time hadn't touched them. Menopause, she insisted, "rudely cuts the woman's life in two." The resulting "discontinuity" is what gives the poor woman an "illusion" of a new life. "It is *another* time that opens before her, so she enters upon it with the fervor of a convert; she is converted to love, to the godly life, to art, to humanity; in these entities she loses herself and magnifies herself. She is dead and risen again, she views the world with an eye that has penetrated the secrets of the beyond, and she thinks she is about to take flight for peaks hitherto unreached.

"But the world has not been changed," de Beauvoir continues rather sourly. (*Whose* world? one wonders.) "The peaks remain inaccessible; the messages received—however brilliantly manifest—are hard to decipher; the inner illuminations fade; before the glass stands a woman who in spite of everything has grown one day older since yesterday."

Lois Banner tells us that by the time de Beauvoir wrote *Coming of Age,* when she was in her sixties, she had become contented with being older. But this was twenty years after *The Second Sex* helped popularize the idea that midlife, for women, was the "dangerous age."

What exactly was it that society, including female intellectuals like Deutsch and de Beauvoir, found so dangerous about women's midlife? Sex, in a word. The idea flourished—-attracting males and females alike—that the middle years brought women a "heightened" sexuality that could drive them to perversity. Unless she were adequately restrained—by marriage or by shame—the menopausal woman risked going sexually berserk.

Pathologizing Midlife Desire

The idea that aging women possess an inappropriate sexuality began showing up at the end of the nineteenth century and continued into the twentieth. Proliferating at the time Helene Deutsch was writing was a sort of anything-could-happen fear that menopause unleashes a voracious sexuality demanding "relief." Deutsch said women this age would halt relationships with their oldest female friends out of "homosexual panic," or fear of becoming lesbians.

Or they would secretly *become* lesbians. (Midlife today seems to bring about more relaxed attitudes toward the possibility of a relationship with another woman. "I guess if it happened I wouldn't kick her out of bed," one heterosexual woman in her fifties, weary of unchosen celibacy, told me.)

Most disruptive of all to the social order, women at midlife were thought to prey lasciviously on younger men. Havelock Ellis, in his influential *Studies in the Psychology of Sex,* said the sex drive was so overwhelming in older women, it could produce "old maid's insanity" in those who had no outlet for it. Older women were sexually aggressive, even more than men, wrote Ellis. Those at greatest risk of being exploited by randy old maids, he wrote, were younger men—and clergy! That was in 1905.

Following Ellis, the notion of a "pathology of desire" in aging women became widely accepted. Physicians located the cause of increased—and potentially perverse—sexuality in the shrinking uterus and diminishing vaginal folds that follow upon menopause. These normal genital changes, Banner tells us in her historical study of sexuality in aging women, were depicted as "repulsive."

Even doctors who didn't actually consider women's midlife sexuality perverse thought that "congestive conditions" in the genitals made desire so unbearable, it drove midlife women to dalliances with younger men.

The horror associated with the idea of older women being sexual with younger men was not confined to the medical profession. Journalists of the day called young men who attended afternoon dances "lounge lizards" and the aging women who pursued them "flapperdames." Women's dancing was a public display of their grotesque erotic interests. Even de Beauvoir, in the 1940s, was taken by this idea of middle-aged excess in females. "Nine out of ten erotomaniacs are women, and these are almost all forty to fifty years old," she wrote in *The Second Sex.*

Of course there was plenty of clinical theory to explain all this sexy behavior. The way Freud saw it, menopause could elicit a reexperiencing of the "castration complex" of early childhood. That is how he accounted for the jealousy experienced by a fifty-year-old woman who came to him suspecting that her husband was having an affair with a younger woman. Nonsense, said Freud, after a consultation lasting several hours; what was going on was this: midlife had reawakened the woman's lifelong sense of inferiority, which came from her belief that her clitoris was only a castrated penis. Her jealousy was a "displacement" for the fact that what she really wanted was sex with her son-in-law—an involvement with his youthful vigor, suggested Freud, that would counteract her waning sense of attractiveness.

Obviously, older women as well as older men are tempted to try to compensate for their waning power by seducing those younger than themselves. Today, midlife women don't repress the fantasy. You hear them in the locker room talking about the gym boys and their cute buns. Not all of them act on the fantasy, though. Deborah Gimmelson did, and lived to tell the tale. "Forget equality—I liked it *on top*," she confessed in the "Hers" column of *The New York Times Magazine,* describing an affair with her fitness trainer at one of those small SoHo gyms catering to the affluent.

Gimmelson's trainer was, of course, good looking. He was also suitably inexperienced. "There is power for a woman involved with a younger, less-educated, open young man—power the way it has always existed for men in similar circumstances," she says.

It was almost as heady as sex, watching the guy "approach his first sushi or the array of silverware in posh restaurants; power in taking him to his first Broadway play, power in introducing him to people he would never meet without *you,* the Provider, the Sophisticate, the Worldly One." Gimmelson gave her lover a dictionary; she felt alive! So what if he'd never heard of Picasso? she said. She could have talked about Schwarzenegger forever. "When he uttered the unacceptable 'I could have went,' I reminded him that 'gone' was the past participle of 'to go.' My god, I thought, I *was* God, or at least involved in a living production of 'Pygmalion.' "

The postscript is that Hunko (or El Fabulo, as Cynthia Heimel once referred to such a creature) left her for another fitness freak, an older woman who offered him superior wines and souped-up motorcycles. And Gimmelson? She changed shrinks and went to a new gym—the moral being, apparently, that ageism can backfire for either gender.

The midlife woman may find that while there's nothing wrong with pursuing a younger man, it may work out better when she isn't on a power trip; *and* if she can hold out for someone with more to share than hot sex and exquisitely defined lats. (On the other hand . . .)

*   *   *

WOMEN continue to be affected, however unconsciously, by the notion of their "perversity." We are afraid of our sexual needs and can fall into the trap of repressing them. The midlife woman who's free and aggressive in her sexuality is, I suspect, the exception rather than the rule.

For women, youthfulness is equated with gender itself. What is "feminine," Maggie Scarf reminded those attending a Harvard-sponsored conference for couples therapists, "is smooth, rounded, unlined and soft." Lose your youth, and you can feel as if you're losing your femininity. Sexual encounters, in such an atmosphere, become potentially humiliating, which is why some women at midlife begin to avoid sex altogether.

"Women often feel ashamed of getting older," Scarf told the therapists. After a lifetime of compliments and flattery from men, they feel the loss of this "gratifying feedback"; the result, she says, can be a blow to their self-esteem.

That blow cropped up time and again in comments that psychologist Ellen Cole heard from women attending the Yale Menopause Clinic. One 55-year-old lawyer said wistfully, "It's not easy to see your chin get double and your waist get thick and see yourself as not sexually attractive."

The challenge for aging women today is to *resist* society's derogatory attitude toward their sexual desires. Women who have been well loved and sexually cherished will find it easier to embrace their sexuality when age begins to take its physical toll. Those who have not had this support may find themselves more than usually vulnerable to the cultural belief that sexual needs in older women are vile.

Those of us with some back-up in challenging society's attitudes toward aging women have a better time of it. Some gay women, for example, believe they are able to escape feeling bad about the ravages of their youth and beauty. "One, if not *the* greatest blessing about being middle-aged dykes is that while heterosexual women are frantically chasing the rainbow of 'lost youth' and are frightened by their loss of 'beauty' and 'sex appeal'—we old dykes are daily growing more comfortable and *accepting* of our aging faces and bodies and are therefore able to see beneath the superficial to the glowing beauty of a mellow soul," one woman told Barbara E. Sang, who did a study of 110 midlife lesbians. (In Sang's group, almost half the women had been heterosexually married at some point in their lives, and almost half had one or more children. Significantly, a quarter of the women experienced their first feelings toward women at midlife.)

Another of Sang's subjects, Robyn Posin, told of learning to love her thighs, her wrinkles, her entire fifty-year-old body. "When I first noticed the dimples appearing in my thighs, I again experienced a reflexive surge of guilt, as though I'd been irresponsible in not being involved in some exercise regime."

Posin's guilt was followed by rage at being "brainwashed into such a response," then grief over the way women are abused into feeling that their aging bodies are a sign of personal failure. As she aged, Posin said, her eyes and heart began to soften, but she also made an effort to raise her own consciousness. "I continued my morning ritual of massaging lotion into my body, being especially loving as I lotioned my thighs. I thanked them for their strength and dependability, for serving my mobility for so long without complaint. I thanked them for enabling me still to delight in my yoga, tai chi and daily wanderings in the canyons."

Sang found that almost all the lesbians in her study (93 percent) liked themselves better at this age, and most (76 percent) felt midlife to be the best time of their lives. They told her they were "more mellow," "better grounded," "less defensive," "kinder, softer, wiser," and "more balanced," and that they "had greater self-knowledge and acceptance of faults." One woman said, "I seem to have less bravado and more feeling of real stature and accomplishment."

Still, not all midlife lesbian women are immune to the stereotypes of aging. Carol, a director who recently returned to Wisconsin after a theater stint in Los Angeles, feels her age as poignantly as any straight woman I interviewed, although she couches her disappointment in the rhetoric of politics. Because gay women live in a society "dominated by white male patriarchy," says Carol, they internalize negative messages about themselves. "The world is made by men, so in the long run it doesn't matter, at certain phases in your life, what the women think. It's the men. It's what *they* think."

I Dream of Chin Hairs

In *Aging in Mass Society,* Jon and C. Davis Hendricks say it is how a woman perceives herself that is most likely to damage her "sexual outlook." That is, "if she believes herself to be unattractive or too old, sex will in all probability become a thing of the past."

Several years after becoming single at fifty, I began to entertain the idea of a new relationship. Sex, without my noticing exactly how or when, had slipped from the back burner to the front. I began dressing with more pizazz when I went out at night, in leggings and sneakers and shorter skirts. I began noticing guys at the bar, men who until then had been mere shadow figures, friezes of joyless drinkers, as I passed into the only slightly brighter light of the café. First, from the smoky haze in the bar, there emerged body parts—a wrist here, a bicep there. Someone's *hair* seemed nice, someone's eyes. On Thursday nights in midwinter, when things in Woodstock slow down to a hibernal halt, Eduardo would play at his keyboard and sing. I would sit in the back of the room at a window overlooking the frozen, moonlit stream and write in my notebook, looking up occasionally to make eyes at him. He made eyes back. For someone who hadn't had so much as a date in two years, going to The Bear on Thursday nights when this guy sang got very interesting. "He couldn't be a day over thirty-four," Willa said, once, as Eduardo ripped into his inimitable version of "Whole Lotta Shakin' Goin' On." "Oh, I'm sure he's in his forties," I replied.

Thirties, forties, what difference did it make? This was fantasyland, after all; did I have to be ashamed of my fantasies?

Apparently I did. Not long after my awareness of the back-burner front-burner switch, I began having dreams marked by yearning and shame. The dreams shocked me. What was going on? I had had plenty of dreams of yearning in the past, but this feeling of being revolted by my own desire was something new.

One night I dreamed of chin hairs. Well, not chin hairs exactly, more like quills—long, yellow-white quills that covered my chin. I wasn't sure whether they belonged on my chin or were some kind of aberration. The worst part was that I was trying to seduce someone in the next room and was worried that he might already have seen the quills and that it was too late. I had no tool for removing them, no tweezers or Klipette, only my fingers. Peering in the mirror, I pulled and pulled on one of the longer ones, determined to get it out, and miraculously I did. But then I saw how many more there were, dozens upon dozens lying flat and thick and long against my chin. I was filled with a kind of frantic fear that I would never be able to keep up with them, and that *he,* waiting in the next room, would find me hideous.

When I remembered the dream in the morning, I was filled with a kind of delight over its obviousness. I was, at the time, plucking chin hairs regularly. It had become a kind of game, watching for them, knowing how to time it. You don't want to overdo because, once plucked, they tend to get coarser. On the other hand, I didn't want a thicket of those little spears shooting up on my chin, glistening, unbeknownst to me, as I leaned toward someone over a candlelit dinner. Thus, with the same persistence with which some go after the elusive little video hedgehog, Sonic, I went after my chin hairs. The trick was to wait until they were long enough to grasp with tweezers' end but not so long as to catch the light and glint menacingly. Sometimes I would notice another woman's chin hairs, and I'd think, "Oh God, doesn't she *know*?"

So, good for me that I saw the connection between my uptightness about hair on my chin and the dream of quills. What about the terror? What about the deep conviction that I was destined to be alone because my body was changing in ways that were hideous and aberrant? What about the fact that I felt hideous and aberrant in the same dream that I felt sexy and yearning?

Just as I was beginning to pass it all off as interesting but not really important, another dream came along to dispel the notion. An old boyfriend I'd had twenty years ago, when I was last single, was very beautiful, a sort of blond version of the dark-eyed Eduardo— very handsome and sweet. I had had a tremendous crush on him but felt, ultimately, as if I weren't attractive enough for him.

So now, in my dream, the boyfriend's back. We are in bed, having just made love, when he asks me to hold my head still at a certain precise angle. I know, in a horrified instant, exactly what it is he wants to see. He has gotten a glimpse of my gray roots and wants to gaze at them full on, to determine the full measure of my deceit. I feel ashamed, and—again—unworthy.

NOT long after this second dream, I began my research on sexuality in midlife women and how it has been perceived. Again and again, those negative words and images came from the mouths of authoritative men, and the authoritative women like de Beauvoir and Deutsch who imitated them—words like *perversion,* "heightened sexuality" (which in any context other than age would seem a good thing), *unbearable, driven to.*

At the same time that authorities were perpetrating these images, the media were making middle-aged women seem pathetic: loveless, shapeless, with nothing to offer anyone, yet fatally attracted to their boy toys. No wonder my attraction to the dark-eyed Eduardo had felt so . . . perverse. I was drawn to him but was pulled back by the feeling that my interest in him was "inappropriate" for a woman my age.

Once, when he'd been gardening (his day job) on the property next door to mine and, seeing me in the yard, had come over to say hello, I smiled, grim-lipped, and then turned on my heel. I felt I had nothing to say to him. Outside the hazy darkness of the café, it was all too real. Simply, I wanted him in my bed, but that old picture painted by Rod Stewart in "Maggie May" stopped me. "The morning sun shining in your face really shows your age." Maggie was a predator, a hot older woman who used the younger man for sex and then kicked him out of bed. That line was how he got back. And it struck terror in my heart when I first heard it, twenty-five years ago.

CHAPTER V

NEW INTIMACIES

*Doing It Again, at Fifty • The Lost Dream of Flying •
A Shift in the Balance of Power • Reinventing a Marriage •
The Great Midlife Escape •
When the Men No Longer Seem Up to the Mark •
Why Marry Again? • Single at Fifty • On Our Own—
and Maybe Forever • Farewell to the Prince*

THE MAMAS ASKED her, one night, how it had happened. How had she gotten lucky enough, at this age, to hook up with Mr. Right?

"Luck has nothing to do with it," said Helen. "You have to really *want* this. You have to be willing to work at it."

Helen had been married twice. Her first marriage had been a disaster of different personalities and different values, of the sort that can happen when you're barely twenty and don't know who you are. The second had been a friendly arrangement that began in her mid-thirties but lacked true intimacy—a situation, Helen recognized on hindsight, with which she'd felt comfortable all her life, although it left her feeling unloved. "You have to understand," she said, "I didn't know, when I met Dan, what it *feels* like to be loved."

DOING IT AGAIN, AT FIFTY

HELEN met Dan through a friend when she was 48. Dan was five years younger and had also been married twice. Her children were grown. Dan didn't have any of his own, although he had a stepson with whom he was much involved. Both were relatively unencumbered and ready for another try. But Helen was acutely conscious of wanting something different—a more intimate, committed relationship than she'd had in the past. "I wanted to be loved, and I wanted to love someone."

Still, six months into this thing, Helen was reeling out all the old defenses, panicked by the idea that if she really wanted this man she had to be vulnerable, to trust. Once, after making the hour's drive up the Thruway to Catskill on a cold winter night, she could see as soon as Dan opened the door that something was up. *Okay,* she wanted to know—demanded, really, in her swaggering, counterphobic style—*what's going on?* Dan brought her inside. "Well," he said, "I am feeling some conflict. I'm not quite ready for this. I'm feeling slightly intruded upon."

What did he *mean*? Hadn't they made a *date*? This was all Helen needed to set her motor running in reverse. "All right, forget it," she said. "I don't need this." And she stormed toward her car, her new boots crunching desperately on the ice.

Dan was no piker. An orthopedic surgeon who'd actually given up a successful practice to become an artist, a sculptor, he'd moved to the small, unchic river town to help support his new work. He had tremendous self-confidence and modesty. He was a lover.

"Where are you going?" he asked, coming up to the car window, which Helen had reluctantly opened.

"What do you mean where am I going? I have to go home."

"Why?"

"What am I going to do if I stay *here*?"

The upset wasn't all Helen's. Dan had problems of his own. He was wrangling with a teenage son of his second wife's, a woman he'd loved deeply but who'd died two years earlier and for whom he still grieved. He was falling in love with Helen, but things weren't all that clear to him yet. Helen wanted him to say he loved her. Helen wanted him to say everything was all right. Helen *didn't* want him to tell her about his conflict. She had never known what to do with conflict, hers or anyone else's.

"He didn't say what I wanted to hear. What he said was, 'I'd like you to stay and slug it out. I'd like us to try and work through this.' "

She couldn't imagine it, hurt as she was, but something told her to try. "'Okay,' I said, 'let's give it a shot.' I got out of the car and went back into his house. And in that moment, something pivotal happened. I allowed myself to start trusting him."

Tears came into her eyes as she remembered.

"I was always half hysterical when it came to men. But I'd never been involved with someone who was smart, who knew himself, who was able to say to me, 'Listen, you're being crazy.' On some level I'd always known I was being crazy. It's what I did to protect myself, to stay safe and unconnected."

What had changed, for Helen, was age. "I was getting close to fifty and knew this was something I really *wanted*. There wasn't that much time left to make it happen. Some people want financial security, or to have a shot at a different kind of work, or they want to know what it's like not to be hungry all the time and stuffing themselves. I wanted to know what it felt like to be loved."

Now she knows. "There's a way that Dan listens to me. There's a way that he looks at me. Feeling that you're loved is almost a physical thing."

But being loved is not a closed book, a fait accompli. They work at it, Helen says, and work hard. What does that mean? "It means staying honest. It means *talking* about it when weeks have gone by when you've cuddled up on the couch watching the tube together at night but haven't had sex. It means saying that that scares you, and what can we do about it?"

Sex is different at this time of life, Helen says. "Also, for me it's new to be sexual with someone I love. It used to be that I had passion with men, but never love. I don't know what it is to have the two together, and I have to get used to that. Negativity used to be what turned me on. The guy would be stomping out the door saying he was leaving, and then sex was all over us, sex was great."

On Helen's fiftieth birthday, there were two presents from Dan. One was a necklace of heavy silver he'd sculpted for her. The other, a thin box he'd wrapped beautifully, housed a marriage certificate awaiting a single signature. His was already on it.

"Sometimes I find my old defenses flaring up, and I want to get all huffy and isolated, but then I look at Dan and say to myself, 'I *love* this guy.' This is something I *want,* this relationship, I want it to be good."

At fifty, for the first time, she knows what good is.

WHEN you're young, you think marriage is going to give you a life. Whether or not the expectation is conscious, marriage is supposed to provide status, emotional and financial support, a network of friends, children, an extended family—in short, everything. But at midlife, husbands and wives begin asking, "What am I *here* for?" It becomes a radical question, one with no ready answer, no "I'm here because I love him, and I want a family and children." At midlife, there are only more questions. Is this situation stimulating? Do I feel loved and appreciated? Does this person help me grow? Do I bring out the best in him? Do I, in fact, even love him?

The reason midlife women are asking these questions now is that they can afford to. With money of their own and children grown, the entire raison d'être of marriage shifts. There is still, of course, love. Love is a reason to stay married. But how many couples remain loving as the decades roll along? In my network of relatives and friends, not many. And for those who do an upheaval is often required if the relationship is going to be rejuvenated. An upheaval—and work.

Those who don't do the work, who accept increasing distance and a kind of selfish pragmatism, will find, inevitably, that their marriages can't go the distance.

THE LOST DREAM OF FLYING

RUTHIE has mixed feelings about being married so long to the same man. "In earlier days people didn't live this long," she says. "You married someone, you died in ten years. Today you marry, your personality evolves over fifteen, twenty, thirty years. You're ready for a different kind of partner."

Ruthie is ready for a different kind of partner, but at 49, the risk can seem greater than the possible rewards. "I weigh it, and I think probably I could never find a person that would be as good to me as Kent is."

What does she mean by "as good"? Mostly that Kent helps support her in a lifestyle to which she could never have aspired, had she been living on her teacher's salary. But the price had been great. For years, he'd paid little attention to her, and often blamed her for whatever went wrong in his own life. While not exactly "abusive" (what does this word *mean*, anyway? she asks), Kent was irritable and sarcastic most of the time. Did she really need this?

Once the kids were on their own, Ruthie filed for a separation. Kent was adamantly against the divorce, sufficiently used to the distance between them to think he could go on that way indefinitely. He wasn't a man who required a great deal of emotional connectedness to feel relatively content. He had his work, his hobbies, and enough money for a comfortable life, but in some unarticulated sense he knew that his "life" had really been created for him by his wife, who kept the home organized (he paid for a maid to help her and thus felt off the hook), made the friends, and "did" the entertaining. The fact that she had been independent enough to ask for a separation after all these years of seeming to depend on him as much as he depended on her annoyed him. But he'd call her bluff. He'd hire a lawyer and make it difficult for her to get anything. He was sure she'd come to her senses.

The procedure dragged on. Ruthie was dying to get out, but her lawyer advised her that to avoid a charge of abandonment she should stay in the house until the divorce came through. Well, she could play the game, but she was damned well going to have her freedom.

For two years, Ruthie had a great time going out to bars, meeting people, drinking, dancing, and dating. The attention she got was thrilling. "I think that if I had been out of the house at that point, the marriage would have ended," she says, now.

But she hadn't left the house, and gradually the idea of staying with Kent began to feel less oppressive. They'd started having some financial problems. Also, astonishingly, Kent had begun psychoanalysis, and his attitude toward her seemed to have softened. Ruthie decided she preferred the security of her marriage to going out to the Holiday Inn on Saturday nights and dancing with younger guys.

The freedom she'd enjoyed when playing at being single had been a fling, a heady experience that told her she was still attractive. But running around with her girlfriends at night hadn't produced any real shift in Ruthie's sense of herself.

Although she's worked full time her whole life and sometimes does things her friends find thrillingly adventurous, like taking flying lessons, Ruthie doesn't experience herself as having any power. "In my home, Kent was always the boss. In the school where I teach, I've always stepped back from power. One year I was made an interim supervisor, and I didn't like it at all."

Power in our culture is very much tied up with having money, Ruthie recognizes. And yet she allows Kent complete control over their finances. She has accepted this with so much equanimity, it's as if she's been hypnotized. Even her paycheck is deposited automatically into "their" checking account, as they continue to call it, although it's actually *his* checking account. To the observer it is all quite obvious; no more flitting about for this woman. Her dancing days are over.

Ruthie has rationalized her husband's power in the relationship. Kent doesn't withhold money, she insists, but actually "gives" her more than he'd spend on himself. On the other hand, she suspects he views her as having financial value to him. When she retires in a couple of years, Ruthie will begin collecting a $30,000-a-year pension. She'll also have insurance covering them both. "I think that's maybe why he wants me to stay," she says.

The future seems anything but rosy. Ruthie and Kent have different ideas about retirement. Kent's passions are sports, reading, and his sizable antique weathervane collection. Ruthie has dreams of extravagant hostessing. "I want to have parties and dance all night and choose flowers at the florist," she says. "It's such a delicious thing, leisure. I never really had much. One reason I loved to be up in the airplane, nobody could call me. I didn't have to iron anyone's shirt, nothing."

She would also like to travel, maybe to the Orient. Kent—are we surprised by now?—doesn't really care for travel. He obsesses about the possibility of getting caught in the middle of some war.

What about the flying she always loved so much? I ask Ruthie.

Since deciding to stick with the marriage, she has begun to think that flying was not that important after all. "If we're talking about building a marriage together, it would be silly for me to have a hobby that separates us," she says. Kent so hates flying, in fact, that she's now decided that his "indulgence" of her hobby was well-nigh noble: "It was like supporting a drug habit for him to pay for my flying."

Ruthie feels she has security in her marriage, if not much else. They've never had a great sex life. Kent tends to look upon sex as a duty. She's consoled herself over the years with a series of emotional affairs or flirtations, which generally end when her "friend" takes up with a younger woman who's free and single. This leaves Ruthie bitter and disappointed: "They always say, 'But you *chose*. You wanted to stay with Kent.' "

Ruthie doesn't feel that she *chose* at all. "Suppose I left Kent," she says, in the line that gives it all away. "I don't know if they would have picked me anyway."

For the safety of being in a familiar relationship, Ruthie has given up her dream of getting free, of using the midlife transition to really begin flying.

A Shift in the Balance of Power

In 1981, Marvin and Bea, in their middle fifties and married thirty years, sought the help of Betty Carter, a therapist and director of the Family Institute of Westchester. What had disturbed this longtime marriage to the point where they'd felt pressed to enter therapy for the first time? A shift in the balance of power.

Marvin was the successful owner of a small business. Bea had never held a job. Now the balance of power in their relationship was being jolted by the eye-opening experiences Bea was having in a women's group she'd joined. They came to Carter after Marvin had upped and purchased a retirement house without consulting his wife. Bea was beside herself.

Carter tells the story in a 1994 article in *The Family Therapy*

Networker, as an example of how she used to misperceive the real issue in relationships like Marvin and Bea's—the issue of equality.

It's an issue that can surface, dramatically, at midlife.

"When I look back at the tapes of those sessions today, it's immediately obvious that Marvin was stonewalling me as well as his wife," Carter writes. Bea cooperated with the therapy, Carter sees clearly in hindsight, while Marvin refused to budge. He hadn't been interested in "negotiation," announcing flatly that he didn't know if he wanted to stay in the marriage if his wife wanted "too much change."

In the approach she used to use when working with couples, Carter had given "tasks" to her clients. She asked Marvin to "think about" whether he'd be willing to try some negotiation instead of making unilateral decisions in his marriage. Bea was asked to consider what role her *anger* played in her marriage and what it would take for her to reduce it. "Think of it," Carter says today, having undergone a major change in her treatment philosophy. "I made separate and equal problems out of his authoritarianism and her anger about it, as if one did not flow directly from the other."

In her article in the *Networker,* Carter describes herself as having buckled under Marvin's thinly veiled threat of divorce. Why? She wanted to save Bea "before she found herself alone and poor." In subsequent sessions she tried to rouse Bea's empathy "for what was labeled 'Marvin's loneliness.' "

But instead of loneliness, what about Marvin's narcissistic isolation, the kind that prevents one person from really responding to another?

When Marvin made it clear that he had no intention of giving up his role as big gun in the relationship, Carter tried to get him to "delegate" some power to Bea. Now Carter recognizes that she'd been validating "the husband's right to own the power"—to choose, or not choose, to let his wife share in it. Fortunately, Carter tells us, Bea's experience in a women's group led her to see she wasn't going to get much help from this brand of "couples therapy." After a few sessions, she and Marvin dropped out.

It isn't enough for therapists to "sensitively explicate" differences in male and female experiences, says Carter. They must recognize that *a fundamental inequality between the sexes* is the real "stone wall against which we are stalled." Theoretically, the field of family therapy has begun to take gender seriously, but in the therapist's office little has changed, Carter says. Therapists still tend to "accommodate the implacable, entrenched position men often take in therapy and try to get traction for change by working through the more pliant woman."

There is no chance for intimacy in a relationship when there's a core inequality that isn't acknowledged—and changed. Such change may be more likely at midlife, as financial and childrearing demands become less pressing. Women are sometimes aghast, in their fifties, to see that they are *still* the ones who are "doing it all," not only earning a living but taking care of the home, doing most of the caretaking of both parents and children, and seeming to receive emotional support more from friends than from husbands. Even their sex lives are subverted because they're too angry and resentful to feel turned on. By the time they reach fifty, these women may feel prepared to say, "Piss or get off the pot. Get *involved* with me and the rest of the family, or who needs you?"

THE social change that has occurred in the last quarter of a century doesn't support the old model of marriage. Today's midlife women are having to discover new forms of intimacy, and, often to rewrite the rules of marriage. Their new self-sufficiency (and the self-sufficiency of their children) allows them to say, "I can pull the wool off my eyes here. I don't have to pretend. I can decide what I need. I can choose what I want."

REINVENTING A MARRIAGE

FOR Alma, it was a third marriage, for Stan a second. They'd been together five years when they began to see that what they were involved in was fundamentally no different from their earlier marriages. But how could this be when *they* were so different, they thought, so much further into maturity?

Alma and Stan, both psychotherapists, committed themselves to renegotiating their midlife marriage. They would gain, for their efforts, a relationship more intimate than any they'd imagined earlier. The challenge was initiated by Alma, who was able to state "from a position of entitlement," as Carter describes it, what she wanted—what in fact she insisted upon.

Alma told me that she finally acknowledged that her husband was a well-disguised Peter Pan, a brilliant but boyish man who wanted it all without having to face any limitations in his life. He wanted the exciting sex he and Alma had had before they married, but he also wanted to be workaholic and remain distanced from his feelings—and thus from her. They were well into their forties at that point and had a young daughter, but Alma decided she wouldn't continue a compromised relationship. When she told her husband, it knocked him over. "Suddenly I had to confront this issue," he told me. "I couldn't have all the work and have my family available to me on an 'as needed' basis. I was told, 'Either you're a full-time father and a full-time husband, or what the hell are you doing here? Make a choice.' "

Friendship and equality are the signposts of the "remarriage" that can take place between midlife partners, if at least one partner is willing to take the risks involved in demanding a redefinition. It was Alma who pushed for a change in the marriage. Approaching fifty was scary to her, but it also made things clearer. She didn't want—and finally felt she could live without—a husband who was hedging his bets emotionally. She had a life of her own, after all—a career, a child, friends. If Stan wasn't going to come through, why should she fake it? She had a good level of self-esteem to begin with, and taking a stand raised it further.

At first Stan resented being pushed. They had bitter fights, and finally a huge crisis broke out. "Before, I'd always run from relationships that demanded what I thought was too much of me," he says. "This time I made a different choice. I really wanted my child and my wife, but facing the limitations that having them created tore my guts out. It absolutely ripped me apart."

Stan says he'd always been "a Don Juan type," frantically interested in pleasing whomever he was with, not so much because he cared about giving pleasure as because he needed to be seen as a great lover.

Miracle of miracles, Stan actually changed. Profoundly. His relationship to his work and his patients changed. Even his relationship to money changed—he worked less and made more.

One of the first things the change in their commitment produced was a heightening of eroticism. Sex, Stan told me, became a marvel to him. The real attachment Alma was demanding broke down his Don Juan defense. "What's entered our contract is honesty," he says. "I can talk about feelings of disappointment, of wanting it to be more passionate between us, and as I'm talking, suddenly I'm feeling more aroused, more excited. Even as I'm speaking about how disappointed I am about missing passion, suddenly passion reveals itself. . . . I had never imagined it could be like this at my age. I had never imagined being able to cry while 'doing it.' "

When partners in a relationship become less self-involved, sex gets better. "What's happened for me," Stan says, "is that the sexuality has warmed. It's become more contactful, more feeling. I used to be too performance-oriented. I had to be a sort of 'great lover,' you know, not a compassionate lover, or an open lover, but a great lover. In that way I didn't ever have to lose control. If I felt sad or tearful in the middle of having a sexual connection, well, that just never used to happen."

The opening up of someone who has been narcissistically cut off and isolated, as Marion Woodman told the Omega Institute Conference, "Conscious Aging," often requires a confrontation with mortality. Such confrontations are likely to occur at midlife, as our parents approach death. Stan's transformation was in part triggered by watching his all powerful father fail. "His health had declined radically in the last three or four years," Stan says. "He looks fragile now. He's lost weight. I just see him shriveling—the shriveling, shrinking man is happening in front of my eyes."

At the same time, Stan has recognized that he doesn't like the man. "I love him as a father," he says, "but I don't like him as a person." His parents' lives were too doomsdayish, he feels. "I think they prepared for old age sixty years ago. They were always saving for 'the day when.' " To do that, to be sure they would never outlive what they had, meant they lived frugally for more than sixty years."

Having come of age in a different economic environment, Stan deals with the same problem in his life by expanding rather than contracting. Though he watches what he makes, he has vastly enlarged his idea of what he's *capable* of making. Paradoxically, as he increased his commitment to his family and cut down on his actual work hours, he has raised his fees and expanded his income. "Even five or six years ago, I had no idea what I was capable of earning. I think I was sort of stuck on a particular number, like fifty thousand. I thought that that was it—that was as much as I could make, as I would ever make. And I discovered that wasn't true."

Becoming more open to his feelings has allowed Stan to escape his old rigidities. This isn't just a superficial change. It has affected even the way he speaks. "I'm pausing more. I want what I say and how I say whatever it is I say to really connect with me before I say it. It's just got to really connect with my soul."

WHAT'S interesting in this marriage is how much personal development occurred when the husband was challenged by a wife strong enough not to settle. Had Stan married a less secure woman, he would likely have continued on his unsatisfying workaholic path.

For Alma, too, getting the kind of relationship she now enjoys has meant giving up certain deeply entrenched fantasies. "I gave away the illusion of the way a marriage was supposed to be," she says. "That was a tremendous turning point in my life, a major transition. But after giving up that illusion, I feel that I can be here, in the relationship with Stan, and not feel like I'm missing something. I always used to wonder if there weren't someone else who'd make me feel better. I don't do that anymore. I know that Stan's not going to do it for me, and that's been a major revelation. That it's *me*, baby."

The Great Midlife Escape

Part of the reason a woman like Alma is free to stand up for what she wants is that women our age today have viable alternatives to traditional marriages. These alternatives exist because we're creating them.

It used to be that those who stayed married fifteen or twenty years or longer could pretty much count on staying married forever. In the late 1950s, only four percent of divorces involved marriages of more than fifteen years. But by the late 1980s, the figure was up to 25 percent. About 16 percent of divorces involved couples who'd been together twenty-five years or more. Today, longevity is no longer a guarantee of permanence. In fact, the chances of an older couple splitting up are rising dramatically.

Marital unhappiness peaks at around the twentieth year, reports Martha Kirkpatrick, M.D., of UCLA Medical School. It's greatest among women in their late forties and early fifties. (Women in this age group, Dr. Kirkpatrick notes, also show the highest use of antidepressant medication, implying a possible causal link between marital unhappiness and depression. It is just as likely, as discussed in Chapter VI, that hormonal changes at midlife trigger depression in some women, which could exacerbate any underlying unhappiness with their marriages.)

Divorce has been rising among people of all ages, but among the middle-aged it's soaring. Since 1978, divorce has increased 50 percent for midlifers between 40 and 65. Among those who are older, it's jumped 35 percent. In 1970, there were almost 1.5 million divorced and still unmarried people between the ages of 40 and 54. By 1991, the number had risen to 6.1 million.

It is women who are seriously beginning to question the usefulness of marriage, fronted by those of us who've moved past youth and into the precious middle years of our lives. Between 1970 and 1988, the rate at which people remarried dropped by more than 40 percent. Chief among those now determined to remain single, *The New York Times* reports, are "the countless divorced middle-aged women, past their child-bearing and child-rearing years, whose indifference to remarriage is propelling a marked shift in the way Americans live."

More and more, midlife women whose long-term marriages have

ended find their new single status exhilarating. (Divorced men, by comparison, miss the caretaking provided by a wife and tend to get back on the marriage-go-round at the first opportunity.)

A 49-year-old department head of a company in California is thrilled about her new postdivorce autonomy. "For the first time in my life," she said, "I could do anything I wanted." Make popcorn for dinner if she felt like it. Slather on the White Linen she'd always preferred to the Chanel No. 5 her husband had insisted on.

After more than twenty years of marriage, Lyn Steinhauer expected to feel lost and lonely when her divorce came through. Instead, she told *New York Times* reporter Jane Gross, she delights in the pleasures of an empty house and a table set for one. Now she comes and goes as she pleases, spends her money the way she wants to, and "flings herself into work with the energy once spent nurturing and negotiating." She has a weekend relationship, which she says she prefers to being with someone full time.

Indeed. "Was marriage always in such danger of becoming unappealing to women that the whole society had to contrive to keep the fiction of its desirability alive and intact?" Carolyn Heilbrun asks provocatively.

WHILE there are many reasons for the plummeting remarriage rate, demographers and sociologists agree that one overrides the others, and this one "contradicts the mildewed stereotype about women desperate to tie the knot and men itching for adventure," as Gross reports. *Women increasingly view marriage as a bad bargain.* With few exceptions, says the *Times* reporter, who interviewed divorced and widowed men and women around the country, the women "viewed marriage as a vise, solitary life as an unexpected pleasure and relationships with men as better in small doses."

Not so the men, who "overwhelmingly suffered for want of regular companionship and the amenities of domestic life."

There was Ray, a 55-year-old millwright, who longs for the days when his wife packed his lunch and mended his pants before he left for his shift at the Detroit Edison power plant. Today Ray has doubts about "women of the 90s," who he imagines wouldn't look after him so well. "Some of these women, it's hooray for me and the heck with the other guy. They don't know how to share."

Bruce, a divorced policy analyst in the General Accounting Office, wishes he still had a wife to "keep the social life running" and tend to "certain little touches."

Unmarried men are often unable to create lives that sustain them, says Frances Goldscheider. "Even when they have enough money, they can't cope."

The isolation that young bachelors may put up with becomes more painful at midlife. Thus, it's not surprising that most divorced men want to remarry. Only 17 percent of those whom psychologist Judith Wallerstein studied in the 1970s felt better after their marriages broke up.

In fact, divorced women are more likely than men to improve the quality of their lives once the marriage is over. "It appears that divorce leads to a wide range of psychological changes and growth among women, but significantly less so among men," Wallerstein reports. She found that 64 percent of divorced women improved psychologically postdivorce, compared with 16 percent of divorced men. Those changes included "a striking rise in self-esteem, a new directness in acknowledging emotional needs and expressing feelings and thoughts, and increased capacity for humor."

Divorced men have three to four times the mortality rate of their married peers, another study shows, while among divorced and married women, the rate is roughly equivalent. And divorced men often die of stress-related causes like drinking, suicide, or accidents, reports Gross, in the *Times*.

The picture she paints, in 1993, contrasts starkly with that of the divorced women whom Wallerstein studied back in the 1970s. In her study, which got a lot of attention when she published her results in the mid-1980s, half of the divorced women were clinically depressed, and they remained depressed for the ten years she followed up on them. They were terrified of living alone, she says, noting that the anxiety was greater among those over forty. Many were "moderately or severely lonely." Although most had friends and were involved in community activities, their social ties didn't seem to alleviate their suffering. They remained furious at their ex-husbands and highly anxious about being the head of the household.

Nonetheless, as anxious as they were, not even these women wanted their marriages back. The reason they'd left, half said, was that they had felt "chronically stifled or demeaned" by their husbands. Ninety percent said they'd become more self-confident after the divorce. They took pride in their new ability to provide for themselves and their children, sometimes against great odds. Of the 40 women in Wallerstein's long-term study, "only one would have opted—and she, reluctantly—for return to the marriage."

Wallerstein's subjects may have been transitional women who were glad to be out of their marriages but were overwhelmed by the stigma against women on their own that still existed in the 1970s and the lack of social support for them. In the 1990s, widows and divorced women seem more engaged, more autonomous, and happier with their new lives. Many express the desire to be intimately involved with a man only if it adds something to lives that they already consider satisfactory.

Arlette Brisson, a widow of 53, says she loves spending time with men, but only if they're good company. A retired vice-president of Tiffany and Co., Brisson says that widowhood places no constraints on her life. "I'm happy to go out with a woman or by myself."

Relationships with women, at this stage, become more important than ever. "I've always had women friends, but now I realize even more that women can be as interesting, or more interesting, than men," says a crack shot, fly fisherwoman, and board member of a New York hospital. "There are so many blobs in pants walking around these days. Unless a man is interesting, intelligent and fun, I'd rather stay home."

Says Dr. Marcella Maxwell, a high-level administrator in public health, "I like men, but it's not as though there's a vacuum in my life." Maxwell has always had a career. When her husband died, "it wasn't as though I had been in his shadow and didn't know what to do," she says, revealing a self-sufficiency that is widening the net of intimate relationships for women this age. "I don't need a man to support me financially and I have no qualms about going somewhere alone or with a woman. I have no desire to remarry and my friends feel the same way."

The difference between midlife women twenty-five years ago and those today is not that they have suddenly lost their romantic illusions. Rather, this generation lost them when they were younger—and took action faster.

Divorced midlife women today don't remarry quickly. The chances are good, in fact, that they won't remarry at all. A divorced woman of fifty has only a 12 percent likelihood of redonning the bridal veil. This isn't due simply to a lack of men. Older women these days have less need to be married and are less willing to settle, says Monica McGoldrick. Having gained their independence, they are wary of entering another arrangement in which they'd be expected to provide cooking and cleaning services. As a 55-year-old accountant with her own business in Washington, D.C., said to me, "I wouldn't mind a nice long-term affair with someone, but I won't wash anyone's socks."

Even divorced women who do remarry don't stay that way for long. Second marriages break up more frequently—and sooner—than first marriages. First marriages make it to an average of seven years. Second marriages make it a measly four.

When the Men No Longer Seem Up to the Mark

The Mamas were hanging out at the bar in the Chinese restaurant, a kind of neutral zone popular with the poststeroid crowd, a place to meet, greet, and denigrate. Connie Chung was up on the TV in the corner doing an exposé on wrinkle fillers. Willa, sipping seltzer, couldn't take her eyes from the screen. "My ex called to say he saw an article in *Investor's Daily* discussing a possible connection between collagen injections and a rare form of autoimmune disease. He said, 'Remember that time you did it in the lines between your eyes?' "

"How could she *be* with Maury Povich?" said Susan, feeling sorry for Connie.

"He has the IQ of a tampon," said Geraldine, the bartender, in disgust.

Catherine said she'd noticed a new dismissiveness toward both tampons and men, now that we were no longer dependent on either.

GERALDINE'S attitude isn't unique; it has overtaken many of us at midlife. Many women today would be content to find men who are simply on the same level intellectually. Hit with a moment of midlife enlightenment, Patricia Volk writes, "One morning you wake up and see his mouth a little open and a string of spittle linking him to his pillow, and you think: How sweet! How vulnerable! I am so, so lucky. So very lucky, the luckiest girl in the world. Another morning you wake up and see that face and spittle and think: Who is this guy?"

Compared with bachelors over forty, single women are more comfortable in intimate relationships and have better skills for making the emotional adjustments required at midlife. Older single men have a hard time getting involved, making demands, or asserting their emotional needs, according to a 1991 study by Charles Walker at the University of Akron. These men are also "rigid," Walker says. They can make good companions, as long as women don't ask for too much. Ask for more than they're capable of giving, however, and these guys will frequently push women away.

That, certainly, is the impression one gets from reading Margo Howard's impressions of midlife dating in a piece she calls "Jerks, Oddballs, and Egomaniacs." Howard describes the trials and tribulations she and her friends have experienced in their attempts to meet any man over forty with more to offer than trousers and a pulse.

"Every woman I know who is not hermetically sealed into her own life has a core group of what I call The Girlfriends," she begins. Howard's girlfriends, who are over forty, found the dating scene in Boston so disappointing, they decided to bag it altogether. Among their complaints are men who "talk too much to be dead but that is the only giveaway." Even the chatty ones are disillusioning, living, Howard complains, "beyond their intellectual means."

She speaks of another "indelicate but nonetheless real" issue of midlife dating—"the number of men who, for reasons of psychological difficulty or electrical circuitry, have hung up their cleats." The Girlfriends, she says, are never quite sure how to greet this information when they encounter it, especially when they aren't given it in advance but are permitted to "discover" it for themselves. The problem, one gathers from Howard, is not that unusual. (Perhaps it's because the men whose cleats are still functioning are out there making sport with women who are much younger.)

In the 1960s, we used to say that there weren't enough smart men. We didn't mean smarter than we were necessarily—just not dumb. The problem developed, I think, because women were being massively educated for the first time. The shortage of smart men followed our generation of women into midlife, and for a reason that's an extension of the earlier one: the more developed women become—professionally, educationally, and financially—the fewer men there are with whom they might form equal partnerships.

As women age, the number of available men of *any* degree of acceptability decreases significantly. One reason is that older men seek out younger women. Then *these* women are left widows. Over 75 percent of men older than 65 are married; only 33 percent of women over 65 are. In the United States, by the year 2000, there'll be two unmarried women for every unmarried man over age 65.

Few men seem able to form relationships with women who are more powerful, wealthier, and more successful than they are. The higher a woman's level of education, studies show, the less likely she is to marry. For every ten women between forty and fifty who've been through college, there are only three single men who are older and better educated.

Having her own money also stands in the way of a woman hooking up with a man. In every age bracket, the higher her income, the fewer a woman's chances of marrying. (For men, it's just the reverse.) This reflects not only the fact that few men are interested in successful, affluent women, but that successful women are able to remain comfortably unmarried, needing neither the financial nor the social support that marriage traditionally was supposed to offer.

Women's waning interest in marriage is "the real revolution" of the last twenty years, says Frances Goldscheider. The reason for the change, she and others believe, is that women are earning significant personal income for the first time in history. And—miracle of miracles—when women have enough money, they do well outside of marriage. "They can support themselves in reasonable style," says Goldscheider. "They don't define themselves around men. And they do well socially because they have friends and bonding skills."

These women are not opposed to relationships with men. They like men, but they want to be involved with them on new terms. Women have status now. They have financial independence, good health, and a dawning recognition that it's possible to be a full person without someone weighing down the mattress on the other side of the bed.

Judith Yaskin, a midlife divorced Superior Court judge in New Jersey, thinks women her age are fleeing their marriages because there was never enough sharing—either of the drudgery or the caretaking. They got stuck in a transition, she says. Women of her generation became liberated in some ways, but maritally they remained enslaved. Not until their marriages dissolved, whether by death or divorce, were they able to see how imprisoned they'd become.

At fifty, Yaskin loves no longer having to ask "permission" to drop two hundred dollars on supplies for her rose garden. Recently, she overheard a man at the nursery say that he was grateful he wasn't *her* husband. Not so grateful as she, she commented dryly.

In the fall of 1992, at the fiftieth anniversary of the American Association of Marriage and Family Therapists, when Sonia Dimidjian participated in a discussion of divorced women called "After the Ball is Over," she noted that married women often make so many daily accommodations they can end up losing themselves. As an example, she told of a client whose husband had come into the kitchen every night to reload the dishwasher because he thought she didn't do it well enough. This had gone on for years.

These day-in, day-out accommodations, says Dimidjian, contribute to a kind of "annihilation of self," as women find in looking back on their marriages. Locked in a neurotic duet with their husbands, they were unable to maintain a sense of who they are.

Widows, too, are hesitant about remarrying, especially those who had successful marriages and have successful careers, says Dr. Meredith Ruch, a clinical sociologist in Princeton, New Jersey. "They don't have anything to prove."

For others, remaining single after a husband dies offers them a chance to "try their wings" and acquire a greater sense of self.

Why Marry Again?

It is in midlife, when the children are grown and women have money—and rooms—of their own, that the inadequacy of marriage in meeting the needs of females is fully revealed. Having become self-sufficient, women are choosing to be single rather than forfeit their independence, says Barbara Foley Wilson, a demographer at the National Center for Health Statistics. "It's hard for men to remarry when women aren't interested."

And increasingly, women aren't interested. "Some married people still ask, 'What keeps you warm at night?'" writes Margo Howard. "They must be kidding. A hot water bottle, of course. It doesn't roll over on you, sock you in a reflex movement, snore, yank the covers, or tell you its troubles."

It is finally beginning to dawn on those who work clinically with women that marriage is not an ideal. "Our message is turning out to be a radical one," Carol Anderson told the same conference that Sonia Dimidjian addressed in 1992. "Here we are as family therapists saying that it isn't so bad to be divorced." Slowly, surely, the traditional tenets of family therapy are beginning to change. "The assumption is that marriage as it is currently constructed is good for women. And we're saying 'We're not so sure,'" says Anderson.

When Anderson, Dimidjian, and Susan Stuart conducted a study of women following divorce, they elicited stories that made them question "the basic assumptions about the family as we know it," Dimidjian told the conference.

Assumptions having to do with women's contentment in being the major caretakers.

Assumptions about marriage as a financial safety net, the most likely environment for child-rearing, self-development, and contentedly growing older.

Divorced women "are *not* willing to give up everything they have just to get married again," says Dimidjian. "They're not desperate. They're not depressed. They feel that their lives are really complete and full on their own." But the biases that most family therapists continue to hold, she warns, "make it difficult even to consider that the state of being single could actually be good for women, could actually help them to lead interesting lives or do creative, vibrant work."

Midlife divorced women, the three researchers found, saw that being single had pushed them onto a path that they would not otherwise have chosen. And though the path was difficult, it led to huge rewards. "It allowed them to finally have the freedom to begin to focus on what they wanted out of life," the researchers observe. "Who they were. Where they wanted to be going. What kinds of things are important to them."

It allowed them "to finally begin creating lives that were self-defined and self-determined."

"I took my maiden name back and I will never give it up again," says 52-year-old Julie, divorced ten years, who's enrolled in a Ph.D. program and has a lover who she's quite pleased doesn't live in. "I'll never be Mrs. Somebody. It's not that I think that's bad. I'm just saying, 'I did that already,' and for me it had certain connotations that I really don't want again."

The "connotations" have to do with feeling stifled, with being forced to "knuckle under," as a 57-year-old teacher of gifted children in Stamford, Connecticut, described it to Jane Gross. Now that she knows how to manage her finances and handle an electric drill, Liz Lockwood says, she'd find it hard "not to wear the pants in the family."

Being single at midlife can allow women to get in touch with parts of themselves they never acknowledged before. "Your role as therapists," Carol Anderson told the family therapists' conference, "is simply to ask questions that help them to think differently, to dare them to dream."

The task may also be to disillusion them, Anderson writes in *Women in Families*. Single women at midlife need to be weaned from the idea that they're temporarily "between men." Clinging to temporariness makes it difficult for them to adjust to reality, to turn to the task of making a life for themselves. Therapists need to help these women "begin to mourn the loss of one way of life, or at least the dream of that way of life," she writes, "and then to move on to develop another."

Single at Fifty

Toward the end of my first analysis I asked my therapist why he'd given me so little encouragement to examine the downside of my relationship with my longtime companion, R. Promptly, without missing so much as a beat, he said he may have been influenced by a "middle-class" belief in marriage.

It was honest, perhaps, but infuriatingly late, considering that the relationship was at that point fifteen years old. It hadn't been a marriage in the legal sense, but my therapist had certainly treated it as one. "Hang in" was the message he'd given me. "You may not do any better" was how I had interpreted it.

And then I turned fifty, and somehow I came to understand that I could very well do better. I could do better by living on my own.

Statistically, after fifteen years together, the odds of my entering another long-term relationship were pretty low, I knew. The specter of a lonely old age—an archetypal fear for single women—rose up to intimidate me. Yet I felt viscerally both my partner's discontent and my own.

Perhaps we disliked the changes that had taken place in each other over the years. He had become a successful businessman, but the things that were of great interest to him never, as it turned out, captured my attention. And although he would have said otherwise,

I'm not sure he liked my being as independent—or as successful—as I had become. It seemed to him that I needed him less. And I *did* need him less, at least in the old way. I spent several years waiting for something to "happen," nursing the delusion that people decide together to split up. Then I realized that if we were going to split up, I would have to make the first move.

I had come to recognize that true intimacy was lacking between us. My analyst used to say, as if reminding me of something I'd forgotten, "But you two are very intimate." He had it wrong. We weren't intimate—we were enmeshed. Most of our time together was spent in reporting to each other in relentless detail the things that had happened during the day. Each of us seemed to feel we were owed a sounding board, even though we would never have taken advantage of other people in this way. Then we stopped even the reporting. I refused to listen, he refused to listen. That left us with a fundamental problem: Neither of us wanted to be used as a sounding board, but both of us wanted to have one. We wanted to be able to ramble on, venting whatever frustrations or confusions accrued during the day. If we could relieve each other's pressure by "listening," it meant we didn't have to think things through on our own.

It's easy for relationships to slide into this kind of mutual dependency. You get lazy and lose your edge. You begin thinking of the other as an extension of yourself rather than as a separate person you respect and admire. You begin to love him not for himself but for his ability to sponge up your discontents.

Oozing into a mushy warm swamp of shared frustrations and withheld emotions is death to intimacy. Couples' tendency to use each other in this way may be the reason so few marriages last indefinitely and still remain happy. We get to the point where we hate the other guy for using us, and the other guy hates us for the same reason. One day you wake up and realize that the two of you have become a mutual exploitation society. Your individuality is at risk. Even now, five years after we separated, I pull back a bit from this summation, wondering, What would "he" think of it? Would his interpretation of the demise of our relationship be different? Am I being fair to him in having my own point of view?

And then the other side of it: *Is it worth being alone to be able to have a point of view?*

That may *seem* like the most important question, because being alone is what we fear most. But it isn't—the most important question is, *Is it worth being in a relationship if one can't be oneself and be loved?* People spend years wriggling around, trying to accommodate each other's needs at the expense of their own growth. Primarily, they're protecting their own wish to be loved, and harboring a belief that they can't have love without giving up something of themselves.

It may be that relationships of intimacy between men and women need rethinking now that women have become financially independent. I have seen this reanalysis occurring among women once the children are grown, and their careers have taken off, and they have money of their own. Suddenly, they undergo a shift in priorities.

ON OUR OWN—AND MAYBE FOREVER

LOSING a spouse is a virtually female experience. Women are four times more likely than men to be widowed, are more likely to be widowed at an earlier age, and are more likely to remain widows with many years of life ahead of them. Nearly two-thirds of women over the age of 65 are widows.

Given women's longer life expectancy, married women can expect to face almost two decades of late-life widowhood. Today, widows in their fifties are growing in number. Each year, almost as many women are widowed between the ages of 55 and 64 as are women over 65.

According to the National Institute on Aging, the likelihood of older widows and divorced women remarrying isn't great, and it declines the older we get. Older men die first or seek younger mates. Only one in four widows remarries within five years. Most remain single for the rest of their lives, typically almost twenty years. "The last phase of life might be called 'for women only,'" McGoldrick says.

Feminist therapists like McGoldrick, Carter, and Anderson are committed to helping women at this age accept aloneness as a rich, viable alternative to being part of a couple.

AT sixty, Sara, a successful psychologist, came to Betty Carter for help. Sara had had a full life and was nobody's fool. Twenty years earlier, her husband had left her to marry his secretary. With three children and little money to support herself, Sara had put herself through a doctoral program and helped all three children through college and graduate school. Her parents were dead, and she felt she'd resolved her relationships with them through therapy and done her grieving. Now she had lots of friends and activities and radiated confidence. Says Carter, "I was beginning to think that perhaps *I* should go into therapy with *her* when she finally told me why she had come."

For five years Sara had been in a dull relationship with Gary, a 65-year-old lawyer, but she was afraid to break it off for fear she wouldn't find someone else. "I love men, I love sex, and I've never been without a steady relationship for long," Sara said. She thought she was too old to find another man. Her sense of aging had been heightened by the recent death of her mother and the birth of a third grandchild.

"This was the kind of case that used to fill me with feelings of helplessness," Carter writes. "What should we work on? How should we define the problem—'getting old'?" The trap for the therapist, says Carter, would be to assume that Sara would be better off with Gary, or *anyone,* rather than being alone. "I took seriously her statement that she needed help to leave him, even though, at her age, her fears of remaining without a man were realistic."

How did Carter deal with the situation?

At the time, Carter was seeing several women patients who, like Sara, were trying to figure out how to get out of a relationship with a man. The therapist realized that these women had no personal problem but rather one caused by their socialization *as women*—"a socialization that clearly defined them as failures if they found themselves without a man for any reason except widowhood in later life." Carter decided to bring all these patients together in group. Perhaps if they could see the universality of their experience, they might see that what was "disturbed" was the socially prescribed idea that a woman has to be with a man if she is going to have any kind of a life.

Besides Sara, there were Annette, a 49-year-old businesswoman whose husband had left her for his secretary; Joan, a jewelry designer trying, at 32, to decide whether or not to accept a proposal for marriage; 50-year-old Gina, a nonpracticing lawyer whose wealthy husband was having an affair; and 36-year-old Marianne, who was seeing Carter with her husband for problems in their marriage.

Although their backgrounds and ages were different what stood out, as each woman talked, was her belief that she couldn't be whole or happy without a man—the belief "that if she did 'the right thing' and worked on her 'personal problems,' the difficulties with finding a man, or keeping a man, would end." Each woman was overwhelmed by her own situation, yet putting the women together paid off, because they were able to view the others more objectively and learn from them. The group took to meeting in regular sessions, and as time went by, they shifted their focus to taking care of themselves, making decisions that would improve their own lives, and concentrating on what they could arrange for their lives, "instead of what they wished others would 'let them' do."

As the women's sense of themselves and their competence strengthened, they moved on with their relationships. Annette decided to divorce her wayward husband and even became convinced it could make a dynamic improvement in her life. Joan decided to accept the marriage proposal, but only after letting her boyfriend know clearly what he could expect from her and what she expected of him. Gina went back to the law, having decided that when her life was better organized, she'd stop putting up with her husband's affair. Marianne learned to stand up to her husband in a way that shifted the balance of power in their relationship.

And Sara? After two years of meeting in the group, Sara broke up with Gary. "As she feared," says Carter, "she didn't meet anyone else, but when she left the group, she was still deeply involved with several peer groups, remained closely attached to her children's families, and was about to organize a travel club." She told Carter, "I'd like to meet a new man, but I wouldn't give up any of my activities for him—he'd have to be willing to fit into my life as much as I would accommodate to his. And if I don't meet anyone—it's not a big deal anymore. I'm not alone in life—I just live alone."

EVEN when you choose to make the break yourself, you can expect the transition to be difficult. You may feel euphoria at first, but it will be followed by a shocked sense of reality.

My own separation took place at the end of December, when my partner was to move out of the house. I thought it best to be away while he was packing his things and taking his hundreds of books down off the shelves. Seizing the moment, I went away for New Year's. I spent three days and nights in an outrageously expensive room in the tower of the Boca Raton Beach and Tennis Club. On New Year's Eve, I got dressed up in black and rhinestones and plunked down a hundred dollars to attend the dinner dance for hotel guests. For the first time in many years, I was alone on this sentimental holiday and—imagine this!—I liked it. I'd gone earlier to the concierge and asked to be put at a table where there would be other single people. (In that group of several hundred, there was one other single, a woman, and as it ended up, we sat at different tables.) I was seated next to a young pediatrician and her husband, and we ate fabulous food and drank very good wine and talked about the problems of crack babies in Dade County. At midnight my new friends and I went onto the dance floor and boogied, and after one long, all-out dance, I took my leave and returned to my room in the tower, feeling quite sated and pleased with myself. It wasn't even one o'clock when I pulled up the covers and turned out the light. New Year's Day dawned as bright as a bell, and I spent it sitting on the beach and writing in my journal while a calypso band played "Red, Red Wine."

Needless to say, things didn't stay at that level forever. When I got home, my books looked amiss on the floor-to-ceiling bookshelves in our sitting room, great dusty gaps yawning where my partner's books had been. Pieces of sculpture—his—were gone; gone, also, the Oriental rugs. The bedroom closet had a bereft look, with scrawny metal hangers left askew on the rod. Most of the furniture, thank God, was mine, and I spent the day after New Year's pushing it around, trying to cover up the bare spots. There were five bedrooms in this house, which seemed suddenly to have developed an echo. Most of the kids' things had long since been taken to furnish their own places. The bedrooms thus had a neutral "guest-room" quality. Only my basement was filled with the accoutrements of family life: cartons of textbooks, clothes dismissed but not discarded, moth-eaten stuffed animals, a ski that had somehow lost its tip. All of this was now mine, since I'd bought my partner's share of the house—mine to own, mine to take care of, and mine, ultimately, to get rid of if I wanted to make room for change.

In the spring I rushed into action, putting up stone walls, sinking hosta, regrading the driveway. I had the driveway circle dug up and reseeded. Then I spent the summer watering it and looking out the window to see if it had turned dry. Early one morning, when the sun was making steam rise from the earth, the house, and the driveway circle, and the lawn all seemed to shimmer and be new, and the project, viewed from the road, as others must have seen it, seemed to have been worth it: as if I had made something new and valuable and permanent. I thought: I have always wanted to live like this, in a house with black shutters and little quarter moons cut out, with silk shirts hanging in the closet, and shoes mounted neatly on rows of metal prongs.

It lasted a day—half a morning, really—and the season that had shimmered so gloriously gave itself up to reality. For all my activity, I had to acknowledge finally the loss of the old dream: white house and picket fence, children's voices, chicken cooking on the stove, dirt and sweat, and the flush of a life lived too exigently ever to be examined. Now there was this gravel driveway, these stone walls, an empty house, and the aching latitude that comes with living by oneself. It was the thing I had spent my very life avoiding, and now it was here.

FAREWELL TO THE PRINCE

"THE heart of the emotional process of divorce is to retrieve one's self from the marriage, that is, give up as finished the hopes, dreams, and expectations that one had invested in the spouse and the marriage, and to reinvest these hopes and expectations in one's self."

Betty Carter is speaking here of a swing-toward-the-self that most of us experience as a major challenge. "This degree of self-direction goes against the grain of everything that women have been raised to believe about themselves."

At midlife, women find that they need to mourn and move beyond old dreams. They feel a need, Dimidjian says, "to leave behind the ideas that there are happily-ever-after endings in life, and that there is a Prince Charming going to come and save you."

SOME of the Mamas had lived years with men without marrying them—without wanting, we thought, that degree of commitment—but, it is obvious now, wanting it desperately, otherwise why would we have stayed so long? What we hadn't wanted was to lose our sense of separateness.

It is easy for a woman to lose that. So we had thought it was better to be maverick; to be, in a certain sense, alone.

Now we *were* alone. "When I see couples out together, I actually feel sorry for them," Willa says, and I feel heartened, thinking of the endless meals with my ex-partner in restaurants, the one endless conversation. "A thousand evenings of vague small talk, blank silences, yawning over the newspaper, retiring at bedtime," as Simone de Beauvoir put it.

I have learned that it is possible to have a life alone—alone with friends, that is, with flowers, with books and magazines stacked on the coffee table, my cats at home on the velvet couch and Satie on the stereo. I have learned that being unmarried doesn't destroy one's sexuality, that living alone can generate new stores of creative energy. It is startling to discover how much depth and complexity lie within.

Still, there are times when I awake in the middle of the night and think, Will being by myself be quite so wonderful when I'm 64? This is frontier stuff, new territory. And once again, in order to get through it, we need to share the experience, to validate one another.

Willa and I are in the living room. A fire is in the fireplace. It doesn't keep the house as warm as the old woodstove that my partner and I had had for many years. Had it been a mistake to opt for the view of the fire instead of the warmth of the stove?

We are, as usual, discussing "the subject." As usual, Willa cuts to the chase. "Do you ever think about hooking up with someone else?" she asks.

"The idea of living with somebody full time . . . I guess my immediate reaction is that it's scary."

"That's not what you want?"

"I'm not sure that *isn't* what I want, either. I don't know. What I *don't* want is to live full time with somebody the way I did in the past. But maybe there's a whole other way of living with somebody."

Of course, we've tiptoed around this subject before. Many times before. More than tiptoed. "If I'm going to have a relationship now," Willa says, with the kind of assertiveness we feel on our better days, "it has to have some real value in my life, not just because 'everybody has one' or whatever. It has to add something. Otherwise I'd rather not have one."

What we want is a full life, however that can be made to happen. And we want to dream our dreams, the ones we never dared dream before. If we get married or remarried, we're afraid we'll slide back into traditional roles of what a "good wife" is supposed to do. We remind ourselves of this. We try to shore up our grit. "I feel like I have to rely on myself," Willa says. "I can't rely on some romantic fantasy about some guy, not that I've ever allowed any guy to support me. But I still had so much invested emotionally, you know. And really, I feel like it's up to me now. I have to create my own sense of fulfillment, my own sense of joy and excitement in life."

"What made that happen?" I asked her.

"Maturity," she says. "It's a maturing process that happens, maybe not to everybody, but it's happening to me. It's part, also, of a spiritual search process. We live in a culture that's always telling us the answer is somewhere outside of ourselves. That the answer is in having more money, or a better body, or a better relationship. And I think that that's not true."

"Do you think that for you, realizing that you no longer have the sexual power you used to have influenced this idea that 'I can't get it from outside myself'?"

"That was definitely a big part of it. When I didn't have it anymore, it made me recognize how addicted I'd gotten to that experience. Somehow I had to adjust, I had to let that one go. And it was very interesting to me because in doing that, in letting it go, I feel like I've also let go of my parents at a deeper level than I ever had before. Somehow it's all tied up. It's like my parents are never going to be the Mommy and Daddy that I always wanted them to be. And I'm never going to find my Prince Charming. And I'm going to have to work hard for what I want, and I'm going to have to put up with frustration. And all of these things, honestly, I think up until recently I just didn't *know*. A big part of me was operating from the place of a child who somehow thought that Mommy and Daddy were out there, that Prince Charming was out there, that things were just going to happen like magic."

"So the magic is gone now?"

"The illusion, the illusion. I'm letting go of it in my life. Now, when things happen that aren't necessarily the way I want them to be, it's easier for me to accept. It's like I'm more willing to just sort of take things as they come."

"What about the *but,* though? You started to say, 'Yeah, I'm disappointed, but . . .' I thought you were going to say, '*But* there's also a payoff.'"

"Well, the payoff is that I'm suffering a lot less. That's the payoff."

THAT year, Willa disengaged herself from the old husband she'd been separated from for years but on whom, in her mind if not in reality, she'd still relied. She sold the old house, the one the kids had grown up in, which was draining her, and for a mere $60,000 bought a charming old vacation house on the river. People thought it was too dark. People said it had no insulation or central heating, and what *could* she be thinking of.

The first contractor who came to make a bid on renovations told her, actually said the words, "This house is a piece of shit." Willa was quite sure that it wasn't. She was quite sure that in spite of the warnings of well-meaning friends, to say nothing of the warnings of her well-meaning ex, she could make this house fulfill her old dream of living and working happily on the water.

She spent an additional $19,000, when all was said and done. Every last dark board was coated four times with white paint. She removed an interior wall and incorporated into the house the huge wraparound porch, whose every muntined window looked out onto the winding river. Insulation was stuffed into each nook and cranny, and a new furnace installed. Willa couldn't believe it. She was in ecstasy. She had done this all by herself.

Of course, the Mamas helped. We did one three-day stint of painting the weekend of Willa's fifty-third birthday. Creedence Clearwater was the music of the day, and there was food and wine. In the late afternoon, the Mamas jumped buck naked off the floating dock that extended into the river, and we swam and splashed one another. It was as if the pristine walls of Willa's new house belonged to us all. It was as if the huge kitchen were a place where *we* would cook (and we would). It was as if *we* would set up our computers and run our business out of a small, precisely shelved room with its window letting in the view.

And of course that was true. Willa felt it, too. It was hers, but it was everyone's.

Most important of all, for midlife women postmarriage, is having a broad social network. "Most single women are not alone," Hicks and Anderson point out in *Women in Families*. Most of them report extensive contacts with relatives, or have a special circle of friends with whom they remain connected for a very long time. These women are actually building nontraditional "families that go beyond our usual idea of what family means," these social scientists think. "When such 'families' work, they may provide even more intimacy, support and love than conjugal families for women in traditional families."

The bond among the Mamas has allowed each of us to get freer, to become what we wanted to become when we were younger. Now, when Willa entered a relationship, she would do it from a place she loved: herself.

HORMONE WARS

"IT WAS AS if the floodgates had opened," said Fiona. "I thought I was going to be washed away with my own blood."

"The task becomes one of trying to restrain the cells," her doctor had told her. "Progestin," he'd announced. "Your body has stopped making it, but you're still making estrogen." Without the opposing effects of progestin, the estrogen was causing the cells of her endometrium to grow. He advised progesterone.

Books Fiona read for checking up on the doctor offered the same strategy. "Shaping up your periods," one called it. "Tidying," said another, as if the thing a woman needed most was to have her bodily functions controlled. But what actually did they mean by all this shaping and tidying?

"No one ever discusses these things with us ahead of time," said Willa. "It's why whatever happens to our bodies always seems like such a first."

Fiona agreed. "I asked my mother what menopause had been like for her. She thought for a moment and said, 'I had one hot flash.' 'That was it?' I said. She said, 'That was it.'"

In the interests of hormonal balance, if not "tidiness," Fiona started taking the progesterone, and before long the "high tide," as

Laurie Anderson so poetically describes it, began to subside. After all the heavy bleeding, Fiona's perimenopausal periods returned to normal. No longer would she be at risk for anemia due to loss of blood. And she would not have to face the hysterectomy dilemma that some heavy-bleeding women are up against.

I began work on this book in 1992, the year menopause came out of the closet. Gail Sheehy had published her famous *Vanity Fair* piece, "The Silent Passage" (her book by the same name was soon to follow), and every midlife woman I knew was talking of little else but the big M. Thank God it was finally out in the open!

But confusing, still, was the fact that we all were experiencing "the change" so differently. It was hard to know what was normal and what wasn't. Some of us had hot flashes, some didn't. Some gained weight, some didn't. Some—like me—found themselves forgetting things, stumbling in their gardens, lying awake at night, eyelids stuck open as if with Krazy Glue.

Menopause is not unlike menstruation, in that no matter what your friends who go through it first tell you, *your* experience is going to be different. At puberty, you and your best buddy discovered that you didn't have the same amount of bleeding or tampon size, the same length of period, the same cramps or bloating or other menstrual or premenstrual symptoms. At menopause, too, the "symptoms" differ from woman to woman—and for the same reason that our experiences of the menses differ.

Estrogen levels begin dropping in the midthirties, making pregnancy less likely. In the early forties, menstrual cycles become shorter and FSH (follicle stimulating hormone) may be elevated; when this is the case, in the words of one gynecological researcher, "the ability to get these women pregnant, even with heroic intervention, is discouraging at best." By then, the perimenopause has begun, and while pregnancy isn't out of the question, it's unlikely. By the late forties, cycles become irregular and periods often produce heavy bleeding. Irregularity is the harbinger of menopause. Some women miss a period or two, and it's all over. For others, the irregularity goes on for a year or longer.

That is but the briefest outline of the menopausal trajectory. Things get more complicated when we contemplate the effects of hormones and other body chemicals on each individual woman. Estrogen alone doesn't act on us at midlife. Who gets hit with hot flashes, insomnia, and mood changes—and when, how severely, and for how long—has to do, in part, with brain neurotransmitters like serotonin. A chemical that requires the presence of estrogen for its metabolism in the brain, serotonin regulates sleep, energy, mood, and libido and is central to our well-being. Women (like men) vary in the amounts of serotonin they have available in the brain. A number of researchers have suggested that women with low serotonin (largely a genetic matter) may become more symptomatic, when their estrogen levels drop off, than those whose serotonin levels are closer to normal.

The *rate* of change is also relevant. Uriel Halbreich, Director of Biobehavioral Research at the State University of New York at Buffalo, thinks the relative speed with which our sex hormone levels change could be *the* determining factor in how symptomatic we become at menopause (and during menstrual cycles, for that matter). In those whose drop-off is gradual and who have sufficient serotonin, there may be *no* overt symptoms. In those whose drop-off is sudden—say, after the ovaries have been removed surgically—symptoms are likely to be pronounced and dramatic.

Between the two extremes lies the middle ground of the menopause spectrum, where everyone else falls. Some, in this group, may find their symptoms mildly discomfiting. Others may be quite symptomatic but, like me, may not at first relate what they're experiencing to menopause. Ultimately, I realized that I'd been being affected by "the change" for years. It was an illuminating moment. So *that's* what that is, I thought, as I began recalling symptom after symptom.

The Big M

It had been a year since my last period when I began to take seriously the sleep problems I'd been having—the loss of energy, libido, even sexual fantasies. Nor could I ignore the fact that my mood was flattened.

A gauntness seemed to have invaded both my face and my psyche. It occurred to me, finally, that low estrogen might be the cause. Then another thought struck: Could the drop-off in estrogen also be causing my difficulty in concentration?

I had been having odd lapses in memory. For a period of six months or so, I stumbled a lot, and in another long period I had a hard time focusing on my work. I felt depressed and anxious and needed frequent naps, in part to make up for the sleep I wasn't getting at night. I can joke, now, about the bleak fantasies on which I'd obsess as I lay awake at night, but at the time I was worried about how long I'd be able to keep on supporting myself. My free-lance income had dropped as my ability to plan and think ahead was compromised. For over two years, I was stuck in this pattern, and it was hard not to think: Is this *it,* the end of my vitality and productivity?

It took me some time to figure out that a menopausal drop in hormone levels might have anything to do with this. No physician I saw was giving me any clues. Some doctors think there's no point in telling women ahead of time about the possible symptoms of menopause. For myself, I would far rather have learned in advance how hormone changes might affect my physical and mental well-being. It would have meant my getting help sooner.

Much of what I was experiencing—the difficulty concentrating, the memory problems, the sleep problems, and the residue of depression that remained even after my thyroid and hemoglobin levels were corrected—would likely improve, I would learn, with hormone replacement therapy.

Once I grasped the degree to which my functioning had been impaired, I determined to become as well as possible. There's no history of breast cancer in my family (more about this connection later), so I began HRT.

Barely a week into the regimen, I no longer had hot flashes and was sleeping better. After several weeks, there were more changes. My face got smoother. Estrogen, whose receptors cluster densely in the skin, was making me look softer (and thus, presumably, younger). More important, my energy level and mood improved. An uncomfortable edginess that had been interfering with my ability to focus when I worked disappeared. There was no doubt that I was feeling better than I had in some time, and feeling well made me feel younger— more energetic, more hopeful. Yet the subject of estrogen and progesterone supplements was getting a great deal of bad press. In downing this "hormone cocktail," as Germaine Greer so disparagingly calls it in *The Change,* was I being potentially self-destructive in the interests merely of feeling, looking, and thinking better?

WHETHER or not midlife women need to have their lowering hormone levels rebalanced has become one of the most hotly debated contemporary health issues. Is there actually such a thing as "estrogen deficiency," and if there is, what are its effects? And even if loss of estrogen—and yes, testosterone!—is bludgeoning women not only during midlife but for years before and after, should doctors be suggesting synthetic supplements whose long-term effects are not yet fully understood?

These questions have become burdensomely difficult to assess, due in part to the warring interests of basic science, social science, holistic or New Age medicine, and academic feminism. Ovarian hormones are at the center of it all. Alternative health experts suggest every conceivable potion to substitute for them, and feminists guard them like prisoners of war, lest the fact that they affect mood, behavior, energy levels, and cognition be used against women. In the meantime, "I don't want to put anything in my body I don't have to" has become the rallying cry of many midlife women, who may, without realizing it, be jeopardizing their health and longevity.

All women are affected by estrogen loss, although not everyone experiences symptoms. The drop-off in sex hormones can affect the quality of life both during the climacteric and long afterward. The effects may be emotional as well as physical. For Shirley Krohn, a midlevel manager of an international engineering firm, the main symptom was tears: abrupt and inexplicable bouts of weeping. At the age of 48, she told *Fortune* magazine for an article, "Menopause and the Working Woman," "I suddenly began crying in the middle of meetings for no apparent reason."

At the time, Krohn says, she "had no clue" that her embarrassing weeping might have something to do with menopausal hormone shifts. Eventually, she took a seven-month leave of absence from work. Now that she understands what was going on, she counsels other menopausal employees, convinced she'd be "much further up the corporate ladder" if she'd been diagnosed earlier. Instead, she says, "I lost confidence."

The fact is, the drop in estrogen that occurs in menopause can disturb sleep, affect sex, alter memory and cognition, and create anxiety and difficulty in concentrating. Even more important, as we shall see, estrogen loss appears to be connected with the progression of certain chronic illnesses in women. Women who take hormone replacement therapy, research has shown, have stronger bones, higher energy levels, lower cholesterol, and intact urogenital tissue. They are much less likely to die of cardiovascular disease or suffer serious debilitation from bone fractures. New studies are revealing, as well, fascinating connections between estrogen, memory, and the ability to think.

Unfortunately, much of the new data and their crucial implications for women's well-being are getting lost in an atmosphere of anti-intellectualism and misguided feminism. Women are wringing their hands over the difficulty of The Decision. Some feel guilty about wanting to feel better. Many view medicine as an evil Big Daddy.

Ironically, the role of ovarian hormones in women's postmenopause lives would not be controversial if scientific advances hadn't made it possible for women to *have* a postmenopause. In 1900, with their average life span being 47 years, few women outlasted their ovarian hormone production. Today, we live half our adult lives after our periods stop. At the beginning of the century, menopause signaled an endpoint in women's lives; now it is viewed as a transition. But transition to what?

To a perfectly "normal" second adulthood without estrogen, some feminists would have it. They worry that to gather menopausal symptoms under the rubric of a disease, or a "deficiency disorder," would provide fodder for discrimination. Menopause certainly is a "natural" phenomenon, and shouldn't be considered an illness. Yet it produces changes in ovarian hormones that interact with other chemicals in the body, and from these otherwise "natural" events, symptoms—and yes, disease—can devolve.

Bias against aging women persists, and is undoubtedly damaging. Yet concern about females being thought incapacitated by their hormones has produced a resistance to "male-dominated" medicine (as feminists describe it) that may be equally damaging. Women die—of heart disease and hip fractures—as a result of not having enough estrogen after menopause. Vaginal and urethral tissues atrophy, inviting infection and making sex less pleasurable. And certain cognitive functions, including memory and the capacity for new learning, are impaired. The question, and there is no simple answer, is: Now that we have such a lengthy postmenopause, how do we improve our well-being and protect our health during these years?

HOT FLASH BLUES

HOT flashes are the notorious outward sign of estrogen drop-off. Some women never have a hot flash, some may be only moderately inconvenienced by the symptom, and some may find cataclysms of temperature change wrecking their sleep and embarrassing them as they try to negotiate corporate buyouts. Researchers at the University of California in Los Angeles found that most hot flashes in a group of women they studied occurred at night, often causing waking. The menopausal women awoke three times as often as the premenopausal women and experienced far less REM sleep—the type necessary for genuine rest. As a result, the UCLA team concluded, menopausal women are more likely to be sleep-deprived.

In those of us who are disturbed by the onset of hot flashes, the question immediately arises, "If I do nothing to stop them, for how long will they continue?" For the majority of women (65 percent) hot flashes occur over a period of one to five years. Another 25 percent have them for six to ten years. Ten percent have hot flashes for ten years or more. For a few—"a significant minority," according to Fredi Kronenberg, Ph.D., a researcher at Columbia University College of Physicians and Surgeons—they last twenty or more years. (Dr. Philip

M. Sarrel reported having seen one woman in her seventies and another in her nineties suffering from sleep disturbances due to hot flashes.)

Kronenberg is one of the world's experts on hot flashes. I heard her speak at a menopause conference, where midlife women were hanging from the rafters in the ballroom of a Ramada Inn in Kingston, New York. Kronenberg was vivid on the subject of flashes. During one, she said, the heart rate can increase as much as twenty-five beats a minute. The body temperature actually falls, because the body is getting rid of heat.

The hypothalamus of the brain controls heart rate, dilation of blood vessels and capillaries and breathing—so-called vasomotor symptoms. A hot flash occurs when the hypothalamus gets its signals mixed. Mistakenly perceiving body temperature as too high, it abruptly triggers cool-down mechanisms. Thus, at the beginning of a hot flash the skin becomes cold and clammy.

The cause of this sudden downward "resetting" of the body's thermostat is unknown. It's assumed that estrogen plays a major role in it, since hot flashes begin around menopause, when estrogen levels drop. The abrupt onset of flashes when ovaries are removed surgically, as well as the relief from flashes with estrogen, appear to support the argument. Still, the exact role of estrogen in this peculiar experience of temperature dysregulation isn't understood.

Considered "severe" are flashes that happen every hour. Four million American women fall into the once-an-hour category, Kronenberg told us. She witnesses a lot of severe flashers because she sees the phenomenon as frequently as possible in order to study it. "I screen very carefully because I don't want to wait twenty-four hours for a flash. As a result, I have a very good group of flashers."

One of the subjects, Kronenberg said, her researchers had named "Old Faithful" because she'd had hourly flashes every day for ten years.

"Quelle horreur!" whispered Fiona, who was attending the conference with me.

It's interesting to note right here that hot flash and other menopausal anecdotes are suspect in some circles. Margaret Morganroth Gullette, writing in *Ms.* magazine in 1993, disparages "the menopause horror story," claiming we'd all be better off if women who were symptomatic just kept their mouths shut. It's those with too much time on their hands who do the complaining anyhow, Gullette implies. For the rest, "so much else is going on that the incident doesn't loom large in their whole life story." Two of the writer's "closest friends passed through this allegedly major marker without mentioning it." Nonetheless, after citing the blissful experience of her two silent friends, Gullette later clobbers the idea of personal anecdotes being used to do the opposite—register loudly and clearly the menopausal symptoms that some women find disturbing.

This reactionary tack is surprisingly common among feminist writers today who don't like women singing the hot flash blues lest they blow the politically correct story that, with rare exceptions, menopause is a breeze. Gullette's article in *Ms.*, called "What, Menopause Again?" and subtitled "A Guide to Cultural Combat," encourages women to fight the "cultural pressures" to reveal all about menopause, magnify it, and make it an "event." "Might real power consist in refusing to join the public discussion?" she asks.

If feminist writers don't like women telling personal anecdotes about menopause, you'd think they'd at least take a look at what science is finding. They don't. Since what science discovers in its studies of menopause isn't always "universal"—that is, experienced by *every* menopausal woman—its information is often deemed meaningless by feminists, if not downright harmful.

The Hormone Connection

In the spring of 1993, the National Institutes of Health convened 250 researchers for a three-day Workshop on Menopause: Current Knowledge and Recommendations for Research. A goal of the conference was to get researchers to look at menopause as a more integrated phenomenon, one that is influenced by both physiology and the social environment. But estrogen and testosterone—what they do, don't do, and might do—definitely were hot spots on the agenda.

Sex hormones influence a great deal more than our reproductive capacities. The big news of the 1990s is that these hormones affect total well-being—mental as well as physical—and should not even be thought of as sex hormones. Indeed, they are so important to women's overall health that the tantalizing question is *why* we should stop producing them halfway through adulthood.

At the NIH conference Wulf H. Utian, M.D., a reproductive endocrinologist at Case Western Reserve University and founder of the North American Menopause Society, put forth a fascinating possible answer: The symptoms women experience when their ovarian hormones shut down may be due to an evolutionary lag; that is, the evolution of the female endocrine system may not have kept up with the rapid life span increase. But according to Utian, some data now suggest that women's physiology may be in the process of adapting, evolving a handy new postmenopausal ovary that eventually will keep us going decades longer in the hormone department.

In the meantime, what are women to do?

A researcher who may have more clinical experience with menopausal women than anyone in the country is Philip Sarrel, M.D., professor of obstetrics and gynecology and psychiatry and past director of the Midlife Study Program at Yale University. (He founded the program in 1978 and has treated and studied some 1600 menopausal women in the intervening years.)

Sarrel has gained enormous knowledge of the many ways in which estrogen contributes to the overall health and well-being of females. "It's how I've spent my life, researching this hormone," he told women attending a meeting at Kingston Hospital in upstate New York, sponsored by Prime Plus Red Hot Mamas, an organization that offers free menopause lectures through the aegis of local hospitals. (Prime Plus Red Hot Mamas is the baby of Karen Giben, a Connecticut woman whose physician, Sarrel, steered her through an early hysterectomy—an experience, she told women attending the upstate lecture, that motivated her to take menopause information on the road.)

Sarrel explained that estradiol, one of several estrogens the ovaries produce, is perhaps the most important for the quality of women's lives. It plays a role in cell function in virtually every part of the body, including especially the vagina, the bladder and urethra, and the breasts. Production of it virtually ceases after menopause. "This single hormonal change," says Sarrel, "probably causes most of the signs and symptoms associated with menopause."

Almost all women in their late forties and many in their early or midforties have a decline in ovarian hormone production, and some of these women experience symptoms, Sarrel told women attending his menopause lecture.

When hormone levels drop, a number of symptoms can appear, including itching and burning, numbness and tingling (usually in the fingertips), formication (a sensation of ants crawling under the skin), and easy bruising. (Skin cells, actually, are big users of estrogen.) Angina (chest pain), shortness of breath, and headaches, including migraines, can be caused by estrogen deficiency—and treated with supplements. Some doctors, Sarrel among them, are in favor of treating women with hormones *during* the perimenopause—that is, without waiting until the periods stop—if tests show the hormone levels to be down and a woman is experiencing discomfort from symptoms.

At the Yale Menopause Clinic, Sarrel noticed that women often don't make the connection between, say, difficulties with maintaining balance and lower estrogen levels. "The loss of body control they are experiencing can conjure fears of undiagnosed disease or senility," he says. (My own stumbling in the garden certainly conjured such fears.)

That estrogen supplements restore balance was first demonstrated in a study of female rats, which were found better able to walk a narrow plank in the estrus phase of their cycles, when estrogen and progesterone levels are high. Moreover, when given estrogen supplements, their performance became even better. When estradiol was implanted directly into the rats' basal ganglia, they pranced down the planks as deftly as acrobats. Feminists often question whether animal studies tell us anything about the experience of humans. In this case, the same effects found in the rats were later found in humans. (At the risk of sounding like a flag-waver, I will say that after estrogen, I could stop worrying about whether I was going to make it from my car to my front door without tripping on the stones lining the walkway.)

Virtually all tissues in the body have estrogen receptors, Dr. Utian reminded the NIH menopause conference, which is why the effects of estrogen loss are so comprehensive. Receptors are specialized parts of cells that let hormones lock in and influence cell activity. Estrogen receptors have been found in mucous membranes, the bladder, the breasts, bones, and skin, and even in the lungs and coronary arteries, which supply the heart muscle with nutrients and oxygen. This is why, when estrogen levels fall, so many different physical and psychological changes can occur.

Of considerable significance to women at midlife and older is the condition of bladder and vaginal tissues, which progressively dry and shrink, the longer they go without estrogen. K-Y or other lubricants may ease the discomfort of dry vaginal tissues, but they are mere topical treatments that do nothing to prevent the atrophying of tissue. The same drying process goes on in the urethra. Slowly but surely, women become vulnerable to bladder infections and sexually transmitted disease. Low estrogen may also cause a decline in an important "mechanical barrier" to the spread of bacteria. "Along the length of the urethra are muscle fibers that help control the flow of urine from the bladder," explains Dr. Morris Notelovitz, founder of the Women's Medical and Diagnostic Center, in Gainesville, Florida. "The muscles are thickest midway up the urethra, where they create a 'pressure zone' that helps contain bacteria in the lower part of the urethra." When estrogen levels drop off, blood flow to the area decreases and muscle tone may weaken, causing urethral pressure to decline and allowing bacteria to migrate up the bladder more easily.

Some women have all the symptoms of bladder infections—frequent urination, urgency, and lower abdominal pressure—with the exception of pain on urination. This "urethral syndrome," says Dr. Notelovitz, is common in women after menopause. Correct diagnosis requires a urinalysis and urine culture, before it can be treated. (A urethroscopy to look inside the urethra may also be needed.) But vulnerability to this syndrome can be reduced by using estrogen, studies show. Estrogen helps thicken the urethral lining, improves blood flow to the area, and improves urethral pressure—all of which help the bladder.

Hormone supplements may also help women avoid the loss of

muscle tone in the urethra that leads to incontinence. ("Menopause is not the final taboo!" announced a woman physician at a menopause support group I attended in Kingston. "Incontinence is the final taboo!") Women have told me that it wasn't until they started to experience urine leaking when they laughed or ran upstairs that they began noticing, in drugstores, the huge signs saying "Incontinence" hanging above aisles with products for dealing with it.

"When laughter causes leaks, can the adult diaper be far behind?" asked Fiona.

Those who prefer to strengthen their urogenital tissues without taking estrogen orally can do so with vaginal estrogen cream.

Hormones and the Brain

Some of the more controversial research on ovarian hormones has to do with their effect on women's behavior and mental capacities. "People have been trying for roughly eight billion years to find a link between women's hormones and their behavior, without success!" exults social psychologist Carol Tavris in *The Mismeasure of Woman*.

Substantial evidence to the contrary was presented at the NIH menopause conference. There, Canadian psychologist Barbara Sherwin gave a "state-of-the-art summary" of research on estrogen's relationship to memory and cognition. The hormone "enhances short-term memory and helps to maintain the capacity for new learning," she said. And it's been definitively established that these improvements in mental functioning are the effect of estrogen working directly on the brain. They are not the result of hot flashes and other symptoms being alleviated.

One of Sherwin's tests measured the number of words that women could recall from a paragraph that had just been read to them. These were women who'd had hysterectomies (average age 45); some were on estrogen therapy, and some were not. Those taking estrogen were able to recall more of the paragraph than the women treated with placebo.

When researchers tested abstract reasoning, they found the same thing. The women given hormones following surgery did better than those who received placebo. "In fact," Sherwin reports, "there was somewhat of an increase in score."

In another study, Sherwin administered a paired associates test (a measure of new learning capacity) and found that in the women who received estrogen, scores were maintained from a pre- to a postoperative period. Conversely, the women who received placebo showed "a significant decrease" in their capacity for new learning.

A few weeks after she spoke at the menopause conference, I went to see Barbara Sherwin at her office on the McGill University campus in Montreal. It was a rainy afternoon in early spring. The school was on holiday, leaving the halls, the foyers, and the little rabbit-hutch rooms where the scientists sit and work quiet. I always forget how visually gray and bland the academic environment is. The brightly lit places are in the minds of those doing work there.

I had been reading Sherwin's papers for over a year before I met her. She has discovered a great deal—looking in places where no one else had looked—about estrogen's relationship to how women think and feel. I knew, because her work is widely cited and from things others in the field told me, that she has done breakthrough work. A slender, rather delicate-looking woman with bright lipstick and short, boyishly coiffed hair, Sherwin looks young, although she has a daughter in her twenties. She welcomed me with sliced fruit, cookies, and fresh coffee. (I couldn't help but reflect that a male scientist would likely not have provided such a spread.) We met in late morning and talked until midafternoon.

Sherwin is co-director of the McGill Menopause Clinic, whose patients she studies and where her research on memory takes place. "One of the things the women will say, spontaneously, when I ask if there are any problems, is 'My memory's gone. It's just awful.' Sometimes their eyes kind of well up with tears when they tell me this." Looking in the literature for a connection between estrogen and memory, Sherwin found that little research had been done, and she decided to do it herself. "Thus far, we've followed surgically menopausal women up to six months postoperatively. We see significant changes in very specific aspects of cognitive functioning. It's primarily short-term verbal memory. It's *not* spatial memory, it's not long-term memory."

Sherwin says she can't emphasize strongly enough that what she's finding isn't "global"—that is, not *all* aspects of cognition and memory are affected by estrogen levels. Nor has what she's found, so far, been shown to have any impact on the current "real world" lives of her subjects, she says. "People aren't losing their jobs because of this, but there *is* a phenomenon in the lab, and it has implications for pathology."

What does this mean? The microeffects of estrogen loss on mid-life memory may be related to the more macromemory failures that can occur in women in later life. Sherwin and others are studying this possibility.

BRUCE McEwen, Ph.D., who is head of the Laboratory of Neuro-endocrinology at Rockefeller Institute in New York City, has done important animal studies showing the stimulating effects of estrogen on nerve cell connections in the brain. "For many people, the idea that hormones would be acting directly on the brain has been perhaps a bit hard to accept," he acknowledged at the NIH conference. He went on to present research that proved just that, and the hormone was estrogen.

In the nucleus of a rat's brain cell is a dense network of axons and dendrites, threadlike fibers through which nerve impulses are conducted. "The mass of nerve cells is really found in the dendrites and axons," he said, illustrating with slides. It's at the end of the dendrites, in tiny little structures called "spines," where connections between nerve cells are actually made.

McEwen's lab had counted the minuscule spines on the dendrites and found that on the afternoon when ovulation takes place, the number of those spines in the female rat soar; then, within only twenty-four hours of ovulation, it drops down again. Catherine Wooley, a graduate student working in McEwen's lab, tried to produce the same increase in dendritic spines by administering estrogen. When the rats' ovaries were removed, those little spines decreased gradually over a period of about six days, McEwen explained. With one swift injection of estradiol, Wooley found the density of those tiny but all-important spines increased "markedly."

"What Dr. McEwen and his lab found is just striking," Barbara Sherwin told me. "The fact is that estrogen can affect the thickness of the neurons, of the dendritic branches. You can show that if you give an adult female estrogen, there's an increase in the thickness of the dendrites. And if you take it away, if you remove the ovaries, the number of dendrites diminishes! And this happens in an area of the brain, in the hippocampus, which we know is critically important for memory."

The estrogen-produced changes in animals' brains that McEwen's lab produced support the controversial, slightly earlier work of another scientist, Doreen Kimura, professor of psychology in the department of clinical neurological sciences at the University of Western Ontario. In the late 1980s, Kimura reported that women's cognitive ability fluctuates with hormone changes in the menstrual cycle. "Most people accept the idea that hormones influence how we behave in explicitly sexual situations," she wrote in *Psychology Today*. But "evidence is growing that sex hormones influence a wider range of behaviors, including problem-solving or intellectual abilities."

Cognitive patterns not only remain sensitive to hormonal fluctuations throughout life, she wrote in *Scientific American* in 1992, "the performance of women on certain tasks [changes] throughout the menstrual cycle as levels of estrogen [go] up or down."

During high-estrogen periods of the menstrual cycle, *or* when women take estrogen at menopause, Kimura has found, performance on some motor skills and cognitive tasks, such as manual dexterity and speeded articulation, is enhanced. Speeded articulation is tested by asking subjects to rapidly recite a tongue twister. The decrease in neural connections made by the dendritic spines, once ovaries stop producing hormones, could affect the brilliance or sluggishness with which one announces, "She sells sea shells by the seashore."

"MEDICALIZATION" is a word made up by feminists to deflate the idea that health, in women, bears a relationship to their reproductive biology. It's a widely accepted term and represents an extremely popular point of view among feminists. The idea that reproductive events might have anything to do with mind and mood is considered especially abhorrent, and produces a kind of self-righteous gloating. "Who cares about tongue twisters anyway?" demanded Carol Tavris, commenting acidly on Kimura's work.

They "don't relate to anything" in real life, said Anne Fausto-Sterling, a Brown professor of medical sciences.

"Absurd," said Harvard professor of biology Ruth Hubbard, denouncing Kimura's reports.

When a reporter asked Kimura what the "real-world" consequences of low estrogen might be for women, she snapped out an unfortunate analogy, Sherwin told me. "Kimura attempted to minimize things by saying that for five days a month a woman might come out of her office building and find herself in the parking lot not remembering exactly where she parked her car that morning. That was an attempt to make light of it, but would *you* want that woman to be president, to have her finger on the nuclear button? It's not minor, forgetting where you parked your car five days a month."

Because her work is in precisely that arena that so agitates some feminists—the effects of sex hormones on women's minds, emotions, and behavior—Sherwin herself has come up against criticism. Yet in virtually every paper she's published, she has taken pains to state that the point of doing research that looks for a relationship between estrogen loss and small shifts in cognitive abilities is *not* to impugn women's capacity to function "in the world" but, rather, to gather data that may lead to important information on pathology that develops later in women's lives. It was her studies documenting small losses in short-term memory in women postmenopause—and their reversal, with estrogen—that led to her later work on the connection between sex hormones and Alzheimer's disease.

Sherwin worries about the effects on women's health of the antibiology position espoused by some feminists: "If, out of some sort of philosophical ideology, you're not going to acknowledge that hormones have profound effects on all kinds of bodily functions, then you can't help but do women a disservice."

"They Got the Uterus, I Got the Degree": Margaret's Story

The biological effects of menopause on women's overall health are a hotly contested terrain in the estrogen wars between feminists and scientists. Objecting to the "medicalization" of menopause, the tendency to see it as a "disease" to be "cured," many feminists deny that menopause affects health—and that estrogen has any beneficial effects at all.

In women whose menopause is surgical—that is, produced by the removal of the ovaries—the instant shutdown of brain chemicals and other hormones can produce sudden, dramatic symptoms: low energy, bleak mood, little interest in sex. Women who lose their ovaries experience all at once what happens to the rest of us gradually, over the course of many years. They have little doubt that something "medical" is going on with menopause.

"My life is now separated into prehysterectomy and posthysterectomy," says Margaret, who at 47 felt too young to be facing this watershed in her life.

A few years earlier, Margaret had felt happy and healthy, enjoying a vital relationship with her second husband. She and Hal had a five-year-old daughter and two young adult children from her first marriage. Hal ran his business, and Margaret worked as executive director of an environmental agency. She was also going to school part time to complete her college education. Life was busy and satisfying, and Margaret had no reason to believe it wouldn't continue that way.

Then, in her forties, something changed. Her periods began to be accompanied by severe stomach pains. Every month the pain worsened. During her premenstrual week, she was edgy and depressed. She consulted several gynecologists, who offered the same mystifying diagnosis: intractable abdominal pain. They also suggested hysterectomy.

Having her ovaries and uterus removed would be comparable to a man having his testicles removed, Margaret felt; in effect, she'd be neutered. "They told me my sex life was going to be the same, but I didn't believe it. I believed something that was deeply important to me was going to change radically, and I was scared."

Margaret wanted someone to come up with a diagnosis that was more concrete than "pain." Finally she went to a university medical center in Albany, where a laparoscopy revealed that she had endometriosis. This doctor, too, prescribed hysterectomy, saying it was the only way to halt the progress of the condition.

Hysterectomy is vastly overprescribed (it is the number-two surgical procedure in the country, after cesarean section). Yet several conditions truly justify the surgery, sophisticated gynecologists agree, and rampant endometriosis is one of them. But for years Margaret was cautious, and she refused to accept the surgery solution until she was going into agony for half of each month, sometimes lying down on the floor of her office with the door locked to keep her staff from seeing. "It's crazy to have something taken out in a crapshoot, just hoping it's the right thing," she says. "What if it's not the right thing? What if it's something else?"

Until she finally had surgery, Margaret didn't know that the endometriosis had invaded her body to the point where her bladder and a section of her intestine might have had to be removed. No one had ever told her that untreated endometriosis could jeopardize other organs.

After the operation, which included the removal of her ovaries (oophorectomy) as well as her uterus (hysterectomy), Margaret was no longer physically in pain, but her emotions and sexuality were another matter. Margaret felt as if she'd been dropped overnight into middle age. "One day I was me, and I was young; and the next day, literally, I wasn't. With my ovaries removed I was barely producing estrogen. My vagina dried up, my skin didn't look so good, my hair lost its sheen and grayed a lot, and my sex drive and energy were cut to nothing."

All of these conditions, fortunately, improved dramatically within weeks after Margaret was put on hormone supplements, three months after surgery.

In the meantime, Margaret was determined to turn the experience into something positive. During the seven weeks following surgery, she completed her bachelor's thesis at home. "They got the uterus," she says proudly, "I got the degree."

When her mood improved and her energy returned with the

estrogen supplements, Margaret went out and landed herself a job as a hospital administrator in charge of development. Now, she says, she has greater status, more power, and a higher income than she's ever had before. She believes that what she went through before, during, and after the hysterectomy gave her new power to take risks. "I'm the same person, but I'm not the same," she says. "There's a whole other part of me that I used to keep submerged and under wraps."

"Playing by the rules," as she'd done for years, Margaret lost the power to stand up for herself and get what she wanted. "You have to be aggressive. At some point you just have to know who you are and accept it."

Today she feels in charge of her life. Much of her go-get-'em drive comes from being pain free for the first time in years. The rest, she thinks, has to do with getting estrogen.

Maintaining a Strong Heart

"There was this beating sensation in my chest like a jackhammer," said Catherine. It had started the winter she turned 52. "The feeling was like a rapidly rolling thunder coming from somewhere inside me. I thought, 'It couldn't be my heart, it's beating too fast.' My daughter said, 'What else could it be, if not your heart?' I would wake from time to time, usually in the hours before dawn, shaken by the pounding. It had a rocking quality, like what happens to my bed sometimes when the washing machine at the end of the hall goes into spin."

Catherine's internist sent her to a cardiologist, who evaluated her as having an occasional early beat, followed by what he described (euphemistically, she thought) as a "superbeat." The cardiologist suggested a beta blocker. Catherine's psychiatrist was not impressed with this diagnosis; he said the cause of it all was anxiety.

Catherine passed on the beta blocker. Eventually she learned that the palpitations were caused neither by a superbeat nor by anxiety but by a normal menopausal drop in her estrogen levels. No one had told her that palpitations and racing heart can be triggered by menopause, so for months she hadn't thought to mention the symptoms to her gynecologist. One week on estrogen therapy, and her spin-cycle tachycardia disappeared.

IT used to be thought that only men were at risk for heart disease—a notably ignorant misconception, since heart disease has been the leading killer of women since 1900. Today, the message on female vulnerability is finally out. Among women between the ages of 45 and 64, one in seven has heart disease. Past 65, the figure soars to one in three.

In 1993, science writer Jane Brody reported in *The New York Times* that nearly half of the 500,000 Americans who died of heart attacks that year would be women, most past menopause. In that same year, Janice Douglas, M.D., director of endocrinology and hypertension at Case Western Reserve Medical School, updated the NIH menopause conference on the statistical trajectory of heart disease in women. "Notice that before the age of forty-five there is negligible death rate due to coronary heart disease, and you see the striking increase in women after the age of forty-five," she said, illustrating the point with a demographic chart. "This continues all the way out to beyond eighty-five years of age."

Women are protected against heart disease before menopause, that is, and exposed terribly afterward. Heart disease afflicts one-third of American women aged 50 to 75, and of those 50 and older it is the number one killer. Could the drop-off in estrogen have anything to do with this phenomenon? scientists finally began to wonder.

The first inkling that estrogen might be useful in promoting female cardiovascular health came from the Harvard University Nurses' Health cohort study, which monitored 48,000 postmenopausal nurses for ten years. During that period, the women on estrogen had 44 percent fewer heart attacks. Their risk of dying from heart disease dropped by 30 percent; indeed, their risk of dying of *any* disease went down 11 percent.

Neither random-sampled nor controlled, the nurses' study has been criticized as methodologically flawed, but its conclusions were nevertheless too striking to dismiss. Fifteen medical centers in the

United States have joined a rigorous five-year study to test the effects of estrogen on postmenopausal women with heart disease. But many scientists are already convinced that women's increased risk for heart disease after menopause is related to their loss of estrogen. "It is clear now that estrogen lack should be considered an important risk factor for cardiovascular disease, *and should be equated equally with other risk factors,*" Janice Douglas told the researchers at the NIH menopause conference (my italics). *Why* estrogen lack is a risk factor, moreover, is becoming increasingly clear.

Cholesterol is known to be a major builder of arterial plaque. Estrogen shrinks plaque, probably because it lowers bad cholesterol and preserves good cholesterol. Cholesterol begins its meteoric rise in women when they hit their midforties (in men it begins to level off at that age), rising, on average, from 120 to 160 before it plateaus in their sixties. A number of studies have shown that estrogen reverses this trend, Douglas reported at the NIH conference. A 1990 study conducted in Notelovitz's clinic found that women taking estrogen supplements experienced a nearly ten percent increase in HDL (good cholesterol), an eight percent drop in LDL (bad cholesterol), and a marked improvement in the ratio of total cholesterol to HDL—all of which help protect against heart disease. Recently, investigators have measured plaque in the arteries of monkeys, given them estrogen, then found a significant decrease in the diameter of the plaque. "The plaque size is directly related to estrogen administration," Dr. Douglas commented. (I envision the original plaque filling up the artery like a plump piece of spaghetti, then shrinking, postestrogen, to the size of angel hair.)

Among those who should seriously consider estrogen, Notelovitz advises, are those with a family history of premature heart disease (female relatives who develop it before sixty and male relatives who develop it before fifty-five), those with high blood cholesterol levels (total cholesterol above 240 milligrams per deciliter of blood), those with high blood pressure (diastolic pressure—the bottom number—above 95), and those who experienced a premature menopause (before forty).

While some may conclude that in their case the risks of estrogen outweigh the benefits, for the majority the greater risk may be in refusing hormones. "Estrogen helps to keep HDL levels high, and available evidence strongly indicates that women who take estrogen replacement hormones after menopause see a 50 percent reduction in their risk of dying from a heart attack or stroke," writes Brody, in *The New York Times*. "Estrogen also seems to help maintain flexibility in artery walls, which otherwise become more rigid with age."

PREVENTING "THE HUMP"

"STICKS and stones will break my bones," little girls chant, "but words will never harm me." What is more likely to harm bones—at least as women get older—is hormone deficiency.

Osteoporosis is a condition in which bone becomes so porous, minimal trauma can break it. Increasing evidence shows that during the first decade after menopause, estrogen deficiency, not aging, is the primary cause of bone loss. Fractures of the forearm and "vertebral crush fracture," in which the vertebrae of the spine are gradually crushed by the weight of the skeleton itself, are the most common results of osteoporosis. Eventually, loss of height and dorsal kyphosis, the dread "dowager's hump," can ensue.

Over the life course, bone mineral density declines dramatically in women—by 40 percent in the lumbar spine and by 58 percent in the femoral neck. In the years right after menopause, the *rate* of loss quadruples. In the first postmenopausal decade, women can lose five to ten percent of bone-sustaining minerals in the spine alone. These losses unquestionably lead to breaks.

In spite of massive evidence connecting estrogen deficiency to osteoporosis, some feminists diminish the problem. In the Boston Women's Collective's *Ourselves Growing Older*, Paula Brown Doress and Diana Laskin Siegal announce with goddesslike certitude, "Most of us who don't take hormones won't develop osteoporosis severely enough to cause fractures." They suggested, instead of hormone supplements, "wearing shoes with rubber soles," the idea being if you can't prevent bone loss, at least do what you can to avoid falling.

Fully 50 percent of women over age 65 will develop fractures due to osteoporosis, according to the National Osteoporosis Foundation. One-third suffer spinal fractures, and 15 percent break their hips. "The problem of osteoporosis in aging women is of staggering proportions," says Leonore C. Huppert, M.D., of the University of Pennsylvania School of Medicine. "Eighty percent of hip fractures are associated with osteoporosis, and 15 to 34% of all patients with hip fractures will die from complications within 6 months of the event," she reported in *Medical Clinics of North America.*

"Of course there are plenty of women around who are, like my mother, seventy-six years old and in very, very good skeletal shape," says Sheryl Sherman, a biologist who organized the NIH menopause conference, and is head of the osteoporosis program at the National Institute of Aging. But determining who's going to remain in good skeletal shape and who isn't is a problem. "We hope the issue will be resolved in some way by creating algorithms to identify those women who are at risk, and those who are likely to go through menopause and old age with minimal fractures," she told me, when I interviewed her.

The high-level math is needed due to the number of variables involved. Bone mass is one; the rate of "bone turnover" is another. "The faster bone turns over in old age, the greater the chance of bone loss," says Sherman. This means, for example, that a woman might be high in skeletal mass but also high in rate of bone turnover. How is *her* risk to be assessed?

Weight-bearing exercise is important, since it places a mechanical load on bone, stimulating it to remodel as it adapts to the stress. Bone is a "fluid" tissue, constantly being broken down and re-formed. Unless bones are repeatedly subjected to stress, the breakdown process outruns the buildup, and bones become porous and weak.

But both calcium and estrogen are also essential in preserving bone mass, and women who think they can forget estrogen because they exercise "could be sadly mistaken," says Morris Notelovitz.

The reason calcium requirements increase postmenopause is that estrogen is used for calcium metabolism. So when estrogen declines, the amount of bioavailable calcium declines as well. All postmenopausal women need 1500 milligrams of calcium a day, but those with a predisposition to osteoporosis are encouraged to take estrogen supplements.

Taking 1500 milligrams of calcium carbonate lowers the fracture rate by 36 percent. Adding vitamin D and sodium fluoride to the regimen reduces the rate by 50 percent and 65 percent respectively. Calcium and estrogen taken together lead to a 78 percent decrease in the fracture rate, while combining all four therapies results in an impressive 94 percent reduction in fractures, compared with untreated controls.

The sooner hormone replacement is begun, the greater is the amount of bone mass that can be conserved, Leonore C. Huppert reports in "Hormonal Replacement Therapy: Benefits, Risks, Doses." If it's begun within three years after the last period, bone mass may actually increase. In order to maintain estrogen's protection against fractures, one must take it indefinitely. "When estrogen therapy is discontinued a rapid loss of bone mineral content occurs, suggesting the need for prolonged, possibly lifelong therapy," Dr. Huppert reports.

It is the long-term use of hormones that causes the most concern about a possible connection between estrogen and cancer.

Tʜᴇ Cᴀɴᴄᴇʀ Qᴜᴇsᴛɪᴏɴ

Iɴ the late 1970s, it was discovered that the rate of cancer of the endometrium, or uterine lining, in American women had gone up ten percent. (What this means is that instead of one woman per thousand contracting the illness, 1.1 per thousand did.) The increase was blamed on the ballyhooing of male doctors praising estrogen to the skies. But it soon developed that the problem lay not in estrogen per se but in the fact that estrogen had been prescribed without progesterone, the sex hormone that goes hand in hand with it in nature. When estrogen is "unopposed" by progesterone, it can promote cell growth of the endometrium, which can lead to cancer. (Estrogen has never been shown to be an *initiator*—a creator of new cancer cells.) British researchers reported in the mid-1970s that using a combination of estrogen and progesterone actually protected the endometrium against cancer. Not only did the risk drop but the incidence of endometrial cancer among women taking both hormones was found to be *less* than that of women taking no hormones.

THE situation with breast cancer, however, is less clear-cut than that with endometrial cancer. Because so many women will develop breast cancer in their lifetime at some point, and because *certain types* of breast cancer may grow faster in women who are on estrogen, the notion of a possible link is important. Some women, though, find it so terrifying they refuse to think about possible benefits of estrogen. As one medical writer said to me, "Why should I take anything that has any link at all to cancer?" It was breast cancer, in particular, that she feared (though she had no family history of it), so much that it made her almost glib. "I think breast cancer is much more important to protect against than heart disease, even though heart disease kills more people. Because you can make lifestyle changes that will lessen your incidence of heart disease, *and* if you die of a heart attack or a stroke when you're seventy-six, so you die. We all have to die of something. I mean, what are we supposed to do? Be young and beautiful, and not have heart disease and not have osteoporosis?"

A more relevant question might be, Does taking estrogen mean that we will die of breast cancer? The answer, at this point, appears to be that it is not likely—at least for women who have no history of breast cancer on their mother's side of the family. Among women who *do* have this history, studies have shown, those who have used postmenopausal hormones have twice the risk than those who have never taken them.

Philip Sarrel told those attending his lecture at Kingston Hospital that meta-analyses documented in the 1990s indicate that women who have no family history of breast cancer have *no* increased risk for breast cancer if they take estrogen. (A meta-analysis is an evaluation of virtually all the good studies done to date on a given subject.) And that was the sophisticated view—until, in June 1995, *The New England Journal of Medicine* published a major new study of breast cancer risk conducted by Dr. Graham Colditz of the Harvard Medical School. Using 122,000 participants of the Harvard Nurses' Health study, researchers designed a new, prospective study (the most rigorous kind, it tracks things as they go rather than relying on retrospective reporting) beginning in 1992. The researchers found the risk of breast cancer among women who were currently taking the hormone *and* had been on it at least five years was increased by about 30 percent. The risk increase was not there in women who'd been taking estrogen less than five years; *and* the risk increase disappeared after women who'd been taking the hormone five years or more stopped taking it. (That is, the risk among past users *or* current users who had been taking hormones for less than five years was similar to that among postmenopausal women who had never taken hormones.) The increased risk associated with five or more years of postmenopausal hormone therapy was greater among older women. The relative risk for women 60 to 64 years old who'd been on estrogen or estrogen and progesterone 5 years or more was 1.7—that is, a 70 percent increase in risk as compared with those who'd never taken hormones. Moreover, adding progesterone to estrogen did not reduce the risk of breast cancer, this study found. Since progesterone added to estrogen unequivocally eradicates any risk increase for endometrial cancer, the researchers think the increased risk for breast cancer may have something to do with the different nature of ductal breast tissues.

Writing in the same issue of the journal, Nancy E. Davidson, M.D., of the Johns Hopkins Oncology Center, said what we need is a prospective assessment of the *net* health effects of estrogen supplements—that is, how much benefit remains after we subtract the increased risk of breast cancer from the increased prevention of heart disease and osteoporosis. The Women's Health Initiative now has such an evaluation underway. In the meantime, Davidson advises women to pay particular attention to their own individual risk factors, "and the relative impact of cardiovascular disease, osteoporotic fractures, and cancer of the breast, colon, and uterus on women's health in general."

Less than a month after the Colditz study of breast cancer was published, a new study published in *The Journal of the American Medical Association* compared some 500 women aged 50 to 64 who had newly diagnosed breast cancer with a similar group of healthy women, and found *no link* between the use of the hormones and breast cancer. "In fact, they found that women who had used hormones for eight years or longer had, if anything, a lower risk of breast cancer than those who had never taken them," *The New York Times* reported, in a front page article on the study.

Dr. Janet Stanford, an epidemiologist at the University of Washington in Seattle and the lead author of the new study, thinks the bottom line is that there is no increased risk of breast cancer in women who use hormone replacement therapy. She thought Colditz's study might have been biased because women taking hormone replacement therapy "are more likely to be in contact with the health care community and more likely to be receiving mammograms and breast exams," with the resulting greater likelihood of a breast cancer diagnosis.

Dr. Colditz, on the other hand, thinks Dr. Stanford's study may have missed the effect because it was smaller.

Dr. Louise Brinton, chief of the environmental studies section at the National Cancer Institute, thinks hormones do increase breast cancer risk. "It's not a huge risk, but it's fairly consistent across studies," she told the *Times*.

"But what about the woman whose parents both died prematurely of heart disease, whose cholesterol level is very high or who has high blood pressure and diabetes?" asks Dr. Nanette Wenger, a cardiologist who is a professor of medicine at the Emory University School of Medicine, in Atlanta. She noted that a woman's chance of developing heart disease at some time after menopause is 31 percent, while her chance of developing breast cancer is 3 percent.

Wenger said the growing body of studies on hormone replacement therapy's effects "is information in development," and as of now, there really is no bottom line. Researchers are trying desperately "to define the women most at risk and those most likely to benefit."

Other risks for breast cancer are smoking, obesity, and, as several studies have suggested, alcohol consumption.

"Women don't think about dying of breast cancer so much as

they think about *getting* it," Sheryl Sherman said to me. "And getting breast cancer is viewed by many women as worse than dying of cardiovascular disease."

Sherman sympathizes with women's concerns about cancer. "I get extremely tired of hearing male physicians talk about an 'irrational fear' of breast cancer," she says. With the risk as high as it is, who can blame women for paying attention—a great deal of attention?

Over an 85-year life span, one woman in eight will develop breast cancer, mostly in the later years. Half or more will be cured of the disease. But when women develop heart disease, they often do not fare well, notes Jane Brody. Women are twice as likely as men to die after a heart attack. Women are also less likely to survive coronary bypass surgery and angioplasty. Again, consider the facts: Heart disease causes five times as many deaths in women as all cancers combined. And heart disease, as we have seen, is far less likely to occur in women who take sex-hormone supplements.

In the summer of 1995, good news was announced for women with a family history of colon cancer. Dr. Polly Newcomb, a cancer epidemiologist at the University of Wisconsin in Madison, found that women using hormone replacement therapy had about half of *the risk of getting colon cancer* of those who didn't receive estrogen replacement. The study was published in July 1995 in *The Journal of the National Cancer Institute*. In an article accompanying the report, Dr. John Potter of the Fred Hutchison Cancer Research Center in Seattle said, "Colon cancer is clearly on the list of conditions against which postmenopausal H.R.T. provides useful protection."

Among women for whom taking estrogen is definitely inadvisable are those who are pregnant or who have undiagnosed genital bleeding, or active thrombophlebitis (inflammation of a vein), or known or suspected tumors of the breast or uterus, or acute liver disease. (Dr. Huppert calls these conditions "absolute contraindications.") Dr. Notelovitz adds to that list those who've had ovarian cancer or a recent heart attack. Women who might need close monitoring if they take hormones, he says, are those with seizure disorders, hypertension, high cholesterol, migraines, endometriosis, gall bladder disease, or previous superficial blood clots in the legs.

Calculating Menopausal Mood

Fiona is in her bookshop. I am at home. We are on the phone, our calculators clicking. I tell her, "I'm doing two point five milligrams of Provera two out of every three days." Click, click, click. "That's, let's see, twenty days a month at two point five, or fifty milligrams a month."

"I'm doing five milligrams eight days a month," Fiona replies.

Click, click, click. "That's only forty milligrams a month!" I exclaim.

"Yeah, but I'm only doing this for a little while. My gynecologist thinks if I build slowly to the maximum dosage, I may be able to get to the right amount of progesterone without having two periods a month."

This is the third time Fiona and I have had this calculator-backed conversation. There appears to be no perfect or side-effect-free formula for how much estrogen and progesterone to take. Certain principles, though, do seem to apply. Women *know* that the less progesterone they take, the better they feel. The question then becomes, "How little progesterone can I get away with and still prevent disease and escape with my endometrium intact?"

There is no question that some women definitely do have mood drops when their estrogen is low, and some do experience mood changes at menopause. (Remember that estrogen levels begin dropping long before periods stop.) One study found that compared with men, women around fifty show increased anxiety, forgetfulness, difficulty in concentration, tiredness, feelings of worthlessness, loss of confidence, and difficulty in making decisions. "These gender differences persisted even when the researchers controlled for age-related life events, such as children leaving home," Barbara Parry of the University of California at San Diego reported at the 1992 symposium of the American Psychiatric Association.

Sonia and John McKinlay, writing in *The Harvard Medical School Mental Health Letter,* have themselves noted that 40 percent of first episodes of depression in women coincide with the menopausal years

(45–55). Barbara Sherwin has found that mood becomes disturbed, in varying degrees, in up to 80 percent of perimenopausal women. The politically divisive question is whether these midlife mood disturbances are brought on by environmental stress, as social scientists like the McKinlays believe, or are sparked by plummeting sex hormones, as biological scientists tend to think. Likely, both biology and environment play a role. It has nevertheless been demonstrated that women are psychologically vulnerable when their levels of estrogen and progesterone shift.

Pregnancy, with its high levels of estrogen, often makes women feel unusually good. But 10 to 15 percent of women develop a major depressive illness after childbirth. Strikingly, many of these women have never been clinically depressed before. "The implication is that something endocrinal or hormonal makes women more sensitive," the noted depression researcher Myrna Weissman said at the 1992 American Psychiatric Association symposium.

"Childbirth is the most radical change in an endocrinal milieu that a human can experience," Barbara Sherwin told me. What makes it radical is the rapidity of the hormone shift. Within five hours of giving birth, a woman's estrogen falls to one-fifth its pregnancy level. It then drops to one-fifth of *this*—even lower than before pregnancy—in the ensuing twenty-four hours. As the estrogen drops, depression sets in—*serious* depression in about 15 percent of women.

The premenstrual week is another time when estrogen levels drop—and women's mood does, too. Some premenstrual women become depressed, irritable, carbohydrate-craving, low in energy, and unable to concentrate—symptoms that vanish as soon as menstruation begins and hormone balance is restored.

"We now realize that estrogen and progesterone directly affect nerve cell functions and thus have profound influences on behavior, mood, and the processing of sensory information—all of which are known to fluctuate during the normal menstrual cycle," write Sally K. Severino, M.D., and Margaret L. Moline, Ph.D., in *Premenstrual Syndrome*.

In a recent study of women taking estrogen and progesterone supplements, Barbara Sherwin found that during the one week each month when they weren't taking the supplements, the women *clearly* had more negative moods, more physical symptoms, and less sexual desire than they did during the weeks when they were taking hormones.

As Sherwin has found, and as many women know from experience, the more progesterone we have in our systems, the worse our mood. Many women go so far as to stop hormone replacement therapy because of the depression, irritability, and loss of desire that can occur when the ratio of estrogen to progesterone gets thrown off.

Some women neutralize these side effects by following a different hormone regimen. Instead of taking estrogen and progesterone cyclically, with the week-long hiatus, they take smaller doses of both hormones every day of the month. This method, which needs to be formulated and monitored by a gynecologist, eliminates premenstrual symptoms like bloating and mood swings. It also, in most cases, stops menstrual bleeding. (As Fiona says, "No more periods and no bad moods—the best of all possible worlds!")

THE year before my periods ended, the bleeding was so heavy, my hemoglobin level was falling. Still, it was many months before anyone suggested a blood count, and by then the level had dropped to a dangerous 8.5. "That's almost transfusion time!" said an internist I went to because—not surprisingly—I had barely enough energy to drag myself out of bed in the morning. Besides the anemia, the internist found, my thyroid was underactive. Once I was put on iron supplements and thyroid medication, things picked right up. My mood improved, my energy returned, and my immune system went back to normal (the thyroid gland regulates the immune system), so that I no longer contracted every cough or flu that came down the pike.

During the late 1980s, one study found that low thyroid was the *likely* culprit in perimenopausal women who felt depressed. Researchers in the United Kingdom did hormone profiles and standard psychiatric interviews with 85 women in the late premenopausal stage. Out of all the hormones the scientists checked—including sex hormones, follicle stimulating hormone, prolactin, and cortisol—the one that correlated most closely with depression was TSH, or thyroid stimulating hormone. TSH, produced in the brain, kicks in when the thyroid gland isn't producing enough of the hormone thyroxine—an impor-tant regulator of the immune system that also affects sleep, mood, and energy levels. The women in the U.K. study who were depressed *all* had underactive thyroids. The researchers were so struck by this find-ing they wondered if low thyroid may actually be the cause of depres-sion that showed up in earlier studies of premenopausal women—women whose thyroid levels hadn't been looked at!

Thyroid chemicals, sex hormones, and mood-regulating brain chemicals like serotonin all interact with and affect one another. If the thyroid isn't functioning properly (as it often does not in midlife women), estrogen and serotonin levels also get thrown off. Thus, while the drop-off in estrogen at menopause may not always in itself produce symptoms, it can contribute by triggering other chemical changes in the body.

Menopausal women with moderate to severe depression will find that the illness doesn't respond to estrogen supplements alone. For these women, psychiatric evaluation is important. Antidepressant medication, which helps the brain metabolize its own serotonin, re-stores normal mood and energy. Recently I have added the an-tidepressant Zoloft to my total midlife regimen, which now includes vitamin B, vitamin C, a calcium, magnesium, and zinc combo, es-trogen and progesterone (I use the daily, noncycling method), and synthroid for my thyroid condition. In the deepest months of winter I add light box exposure. And of course I exercise—weight lifting and step aerobics. This is what it takes for me to feel well—energetic and optimistic, with a well-functioning immune system that keeps me from getting sick. My doctor tells me that in the spring I may be able to stop taking the Zoloft and rely only on the light box (a powerful antidepressant). In the meantime, I'm not complaining. I feel "bal-anced" for the first time in five years.

Losing It: The Ultimate Illness

"We now know," Barbara Sherwin told me, "there's a three-to-one female-to-male ratio in the prevalence of Alzheimer's disease in the world that cuts across all cultures, all countries. It's true in Russia, it's true in Finland, it's true in Brooklyn." With such a huge epidemiological gap between genders, looking at the possible role of sex hormones in this disease, she believed, was only good science.

By the early 1990s, Sherwin's lab was not only showing that women *lose* memory after hysterectomies, it was also showing that women who take estrogen, postsurgery, don't. "It made sense for us to ask, Might estrogen even retard the deterioration that is part of *any* degenerative disease?" Sherwin said, the day we talked. "Even if we were only able to use it to hold the line, with Alzheimer's, that would be valuable."

Sherwin proceeded to another intriguing piece of research. This time she studied healthy postmenopausal women from a broad socio-economic range living in the community, rather than women who'd come to her clinic with menopausal complaints. None were on estrogen therapy at the time, or in psychiatric treatment, and they were matched with control subjects for age, social, and education status. Would these women show a change in memory abilities after going on estrogen? Sherwin wanted to find out.

They did indeed. "Estrogen users recalled more information from standardized short stories read to them, both immediately and following a 30-minute delay," she reported in *Obstetrics and Gynecology*. (Other cognitive functions tested in this study seemed to be unaffected by the estrogen, suggesting once again that it has a *specific*, not a global effect on cognition.)

Other scientists were at work on estrogen and Alzheimer's as well. In the fall of 1993, Dr. Victor Henderson of the University of Southern California announced the results of his study of 2,418 women. "We found that women who had used estrogen replacement therapy were forty percent less likely to have Alzheimer's and related dementias compared to women who had not used estrogen."

"Most people, including doctors, are not aware that the brain is a major target of estrogen," said Dr. Dominique Toran-Allerand, a developmental neuroscientist at Columbia University College of Physicians and Surgeons in New York.

When Toran-Allerand applied estrogen to neurons located in the cerebral cortex of rat brains, she found that the neurons began filling up with the chemical messages needed to manufacture nerve growth hormone. Subsequently, she and her colleagues reported in *The Journal of Neuroscience,* in February 1994, that the hormone may exert its influence by making neurons more sensitive to the stimulus of nerve growth factor, a protein thought to play a role in the growth and sustenance of dendrites and axon. These filaments, explains Natalie Angier in *The New York Times,* "which extend from the body of a nerve cell like arms extending from an octopus, convey signals from the nerve cell to its neighbors; they are the wiring that allows neurons to communicate."

Bruce McEwen thinks estrogen's effects on the brain extend well beyond its involvement with nerve growth factor. He and his colleagues have found that estrogen also spurs the growth of an important brain enzyme called "choline acetyltransferase." This enzyme is needed to synthesize acetylcholine, the substance that allows messages to pass from one neuron to the next in the hippocampus, "the throne of memory."

It's been known for some time that people with Alzheimer's have 60 to 90 percent less choline acetyltransferase than those who don't have the disease. "That enzyme deficit could explain at least some of the forgetfulness, cognitive impairments and psychosis associated with Alzheimer's," reports Angier. "And lack of estrogen could be one reason choline acetyltransferase levels fall in the first place."

"Neuroscientists have expressed relief that at last the world may begin to appreciate the importance of the hormone to the health of the human brain," wrote Angier, a year after I interviewed Sherwin. Her article summarized new research—including Sherwin's—suggesting that estrogen operates in brain cells *throughout life,* assuring production of critical enzymes and "maintaining the densest possible mesh of fibers connecting one nerve cell to the next, the kind of synaptic complexity that characterizes a thinking, remembering, robust brain."

Testosterone Wars?

Not surprisingly, sex-hormone changes affect the cognitive abilities of males as well. Doreen Kimura of the University of Western Ontario reported last year in *Scientific American* that she had observed seasonal fluctuations in spatial ability in men: "Their performance improved in spring, when testosterone levels are lower."

Though males experience a more gradual drop in sex hormones than women, between the ages of 48 and 70 their testosterone levels may fall off by as much as 30 to 40 percent. Some researchers believe these drops produce increased body fat and lowered bone density. Testosterone loss may also affect men's mood and lower their energy levels, assertiveness, and concentration.

The NIH is currently researching whether hormone replacement therapy can help fend off bone loss, frailty, and depression in males. During the early 1990s, several scientists conducted pilot studies of the effects of testosterone supplementation in men over 54 years old with low-to-normal testosterone levels. "The results were generally positive, including a gain in lean body mass and strength, a possible decline in bone resorption (with the potential to reverse or improve frailty), an increase in reported sexual desire and activity, and better spatial cognition and word memory," John M. Hoberman and Charles E. Yesalis reported in *Scientific American* early in 1995.

As it turns out, testosterone appears not to be "the dread hormone of aggression," Angier wrote in the *Times*, in June 1995. "It may not be the substance that drives men to behave with quintessential guyness, to posture, push, yelp, belch, punch and play air-guitar. If anything, this most freighted of hormones may be a source of very different sensations: calmness, happiness, and friendliness, for example."

What was the cause of this front page exhilaration? At a meeting of the Endocrine Society, researchers had announced that it was a *deficiency* of testosterone that could lead to the negative behaviors that until now have been thought to occur when levels of the hormone are too high. Dr. Christiana Wang, of the University of California at Los Angeles, and her colleagues studied a group of hypogonadal, or low-testosterone men. These guys weren't feeling passive, depressed, or timid, as might have been expected with a testosterone deficiency. Instead they described feeling edgy, angry, irritable, and aggressive. *And,* when treated with testosterone, they evened out, enjoying a marked increase in well-being.

"Testosterone therapy also appears to give men and women more energy, vim, the desire to leap out of bed in the morning and embrace the demands of the day with can-do concentration," says Angier. "That zestiness is not the same as aggression, which if anything is often accompanied by poor concentration and underlying malaise, researchers said."

Another fascinating new study indicates that the big hormone in the aggression department is estrogen! Researchers in Pennsylvania compared the effects of giving estrogen therapy to girls with delayed onset puberty to giving testosterone to boys with delayed onset puberty. Remarkably, the girls showed earlier and larger increases in aggression with their estrogen beefed up than did the boys with added testosterone—at least until the boys received their last and highest dose of the hormone.

The researchers proposed that for both sexes, the cause of the teen-age spike in aggression is estrogen. How could this be? There's some trickiness here. Scientists are just beginning to understand that most effects of testosterone on the brain, paradoxically, are estrogenic in nature. That is because the brain is rich in an enzyme that converts testosterone into estrogen. The converted hormone then acts on the nerve cells of the brain through estrogen receptors. Male brains also have some receptors for testosterone, but far fewer receptors than they have for estrogen! Thus, in both boys and girls experiencing the hormonal spikes of adolescence, "the influence of either hormone on the brain and behavior probably works its dark art as estrogen," Angier reports. "In the Pennsylvania study, the girls may have had a jump on aggressive behavior over the boys because they were given direct injections of estrogen and therefore their brains did not need to go through the work of converting testosterone to estrogen."

The centrality of the brain's estrogen receptors to aggressive behavior was highlighted by a new study of male mice that were genetically altered so that they lacked nearly all estrogen receptors. Their behavior was vividly different than normal males whose estrogen receptors are intact; these respond to intruders in their territory with violent attacks. The estrogen deficient males reacted tepidly to newcomers, if at all. Significantly, these altered males had all their testosterone receptors intact. *It was only the ability of their brains to metabolize estrogen that was deficient!*

There are no studies yet on the behavior of female mice lacking estrogen receptors. Until then, Angier offers a new hormonal cliché to explain aggression: "The estrogen was so thick you couldn't beat it down with a rolling pin."

It is possible that the more overt symptoms produced by the abrupt shifts in women's hormones provoked scientists to investigate the effects of female hormone loss before studying the effects on men of losing testosterone. But men's turn is coming—not only for hormone supplementation (a testosterone patch is on the drawing board) but for a raging debate on whether male hormone deficiency exists.

"Mass testosterone therapy could become standard medical practice within a decade," Hoberman and Yesalis believe. Already the Hormonal Healthcare Center in London is administering testosterone injections to hundreds of men regardless of age. "Indeed, aging is increasingly being viewed as a medical problem," observe Hoberman and Yesalis, "and this shift is leading to the recognition of a 'male menopause' as treatable as its female counterpart."

In fact, the testosterone wars have already begun. "I don't believe in the male midlife crisis," says Dr. John B. McKinlay, an epidemiologist at Boston University. Nevertheless, he's convinced such a syndrome will exist by the year 2000. Why? "There's a very strong interest in treating aging men for profit, just as there is for aging women."

Fear of Medicine

Distrust of medicine and reverence for what is "natural" has closed the minds of many women to the importance of ovarian hormones to health. Feminists attack medicine for its laggardliness on women's health research, as well as for the laxity and condescension of clinicians. But feminist resistance also comes from what Barbara Sherwin calls "paranoia." The misguided feminist view, she says, is that "if industry has anything to do with it, if male gynecologists have anything to do with it, then it can't be good."

While interviewing women for this book, I was surprised by how often they expressed the conviction that they are better able than their doctors to determine adequate health care—particularly for gynecological health. Some feel bolstered by holistic alternatives. One woman had refused to have a lumpectomy, even though her doctor, suspecting malignancy, recommended it. This woman had undergone the same procedure a few years earlier, and when her biopsy was negative, she felt she'd wasted her money. "This time I'm going to live with my tumor and treat it holistically," she told me, by which she meant injecting herself regularly with mistletoe extract.

Women today are responding to hyped warnings against a "propaganda assault" favoring "medically problematic 'hormone replacement therapy,' " as one journalist recently put it. But actually fewer women are taking estrogen than ought to, in part because of caveats from uninformed writers. Only about one menopausal woman in seven takes hormone replacement. And, according to the NIH, 60 percent of those who start estrogen stop it—even though they *feel* overwhelmingly better—within six months. Their main reason for quitting? They are worried about safety. (The second reason, alas, is their concern about the minor weight gain estrogen causes in some women. In general, women on estrogen tend to be thinner than those who are not on it, although this difference may be due to lifestyle.)

Estrogen has a relationship to women's wellness *now,* in our forties and fifties. This is an important fact to grasp, because how well we feel or don't feel affects our capacity to take advantage of the opportunities available to us at this time of life. Women who don't feel well aren't able to think positively about and plan for their futures. They tend to become resigned, "making do" with less energy, less libido, and less hope, mistakenly believing that it is *age* that is striking them down rather than estrogen-related conditions that are often treatable.

CHAPTER VII

LOVE IN THE AFTERNOON

SEX AND THE MENOPAUSAL WOMAN

When Physiology Intervenes • The Vagina at Menopause •
Hormones and Desire • Vive la Testosterone Différence! •
The PC Muscles: Strengthening Our Possibilities •
Sex and the Midlife Male • The Powerful Potential of Fifties Sex •
Playing It Safe • Making Choices Without Repressing Our Sexuality

"I TRY TO KEEP the lights dim. I try to leave on as many clothes as possible for as long as possible."

Catherine and Willa laugh. Willa is reviewing the vulnerabilities of sex for the single midlife woman. Catherine, who feels like a girl it's been so long since she's been intimate with a man, says, "Give me a for instance."

"Like we'll be in bed doing it, and I'll have a shirt on or something."

"Really?"

"Yeah. I don't feel like I have to take all my clothes off just to have intercourse."

"Men never *ask* you to take your clothes off?"

"If they're getting excited enough about it, they may not even care."

"Does that mean it's up to you to get them so excited they won't notice if your clothes are on or off?"

"Sometimes, you know, it's sort of more erotic if you're getting really into it while you still have clothes on."

"Yes, but are you *conscious* of all this while you're—I mean, is this something that's sticking in your mind, that you have to get the guy hot enough so he doesn't notice the clothes?"

"I'm definitely conscious of wanting them not to notice my body."

"Forget *body*—you don't want them noticing your clothes are still on. How could they notice your body? They can't *see* your body!"

Catherine is beginning to get that thank-God-I'm-past-all-this feeling, although she knows it's defensive. And Willa, in describing her situation, begins to glimpse how trapped she feels. "I mean, it's ridiculous. If a guy wants me to get on top, I'm worried about my stomach hanging over him."

"Your stomach?" says Catherine. "What about your face?"

Inadvertently, or perhaps out of some deep wish to self-destruct, Catherine had recently leaned over a hand mirror lying on a chair in her bedroom and watched the features of her face fall forward as if she were in a fun house. *Is this what a man would see if she were on top?* "This is an illusion, something optical, it's not *you*," she'd told herself, trying not to become hysterical. But it was her. Mirrors don't lie.

"It's not that I *have* to be in the missionary position," Willa continues, unable to let it go. "It's just that my stomach looks flat when I'm on my back."

"Right. And your face," Catherine adds.

"Probably it's the main reason my sex life is diminishing—all these negative feelings about my body. And my face."

Catherine's sex life has diminished to zero. Can she fault Willa for behaving like an obsessed teenager in a game in which she, Catherine, isn't even a player?

Catherine and Willa's conversation is reflective of yet another way in which women in their fifties today are different from earlier generations of women at this age. At the vanguard of the sexual revolution in our thirties, we have had far more sexual experience than women who came before us. It affects the way we look at our sexual futures. In a word, we expect to keep on having sex for years to come. We may even look forward to having better sex than we had when we were younger, because of who we've grown into: ripe, mature, self-knowing, and compassionate women.

Still, at this time of life we have anxieties about the physiological changes that begin affecting our sexual response. The cultural taboo against sexuality in older women helps keep us in the dark about normal midlife sexual changes. This is something to fight, as we have fought against so many taboos that limit our capacity to have full lives. We have another Choice Point here—a place where our own ability to decide and to act can affect, tremendously, the quality of our lives, both now and in the future. Women who want to be Red Hot Mamas in their sixties, seventies, and eighties can ameliorate, work with, or even prevent the sexual changes triggered by menopause.

When Physiology Intervenes

"There's still an orgasm, but it's different now. It's not so intense, not so deeply feeling. It takes a longer time, and lots of stimulation," said a woman visiting the Yale Menopause Clinic.

Many women do report a lowered orgasmic response after menopause. Forty percent of those surveyed by psychologist Ellen Cole, at the Yale Clinic, said they experienced some change: It took them longer to get there, and/or their orgasms were less intense.

Just as our other reflexes slow down as we age, so too do our sexual reflexes. Arousal, that flooding of sexual feelings we call "turning on," with its accompanying vaginal lubrication, doesn't always occur with the first touch of a hand on our breast or a single kiss on the neck, as it did when we were teenagers.

"It takes me fifteen minutes just to build to an intensity that used to take, it seemed, seconds," a woman told Cole.

If we don't *know* that this slower start-up is normal at midlife, we may panic, thinking, "My God, I've lost it. I'm not sexy anymore." That anxiety can further suppress sexual response; it's hard to feel distressed and sexy at the same time. On the other hand, if we *expect* a slower start off the blocks, we can relax into sexual foreplay, knowing that it will still get us to the same place.

William Masters and Virginia Johnson, the pioneer researchers on human sexuality, wrote in *Human Sexual Response* that women of virtually any age are fully capable of having orgasms, particularly when they are regularly exposed to effective sexual stimulation: "In short, there is no time limit drawn by advancing years to female sexuality."

"Granted good health," says Dr. Wardell Pomeroy, a colleague of sex researcher Alfred Kinsey, women who are getting older "can have orgasms or multiple orgasms as well as they did in their forties and fifties, *which is their peak.*"

In a survey of 800 American men and women conducted by Bernard Starr and Marcella Weiner, 87 percent of the female respondents said that sex after menopause was the same or better. The majority of them were sexually active.

HOWEVER, a diminishment of orgasm may occur at menopause due to less blood flowing to the vagina. In younger women the outer third of the vagina becomes swollen with blood as orgasm approaches. After menopause, when less blood gets to the area, sexual arousal creates less genital congestion, or swelling. What Masters and Johnson call "the orgasmic platform" isn't as great, and the resulting orgasm isn't either. Older women also experience fewer vaginal contractions during orgasm, down to three to five, from five to ten in youth.

For some of the patients at the Yale clinic, the orgasm problem was clearly clitoral. "My clitoris has become desensitized, and there's very little reaction," said one. Such complaints are often due to atrophy. Low estrogen can eventually shrink the clitoris—although, as with so many estrogen-related changes, this, too, is reversible with treatment.

Women whose orgasms become smaller or less frequent may find that hormone replacement therapy helps. In Sarrel's London Menopause Study, one in four women were no longer able to have orgasms after menopause, but with hormone replacement therapy, 80 percent became orgasmic again.

In fact, women on hormone replacement therapy are more likely to have a strong interest in sex, to reach orgasm, to rate their sex lives as "enjoyable," and to masturbate, Sarrel reports. Not surprisingly, given all that, they are also twice as likely to be involved in a sexual relationship as women who are not on HRT.

Sarrel's London Menopause Study set out to discover what the women who reported having no sexual problems had in common. What he found is intriguing. One out of three of the sex-is-great women had a new partner. Having someone new seems to revitalize sexual interest, and that, in turn, may keep other sexual problems at bay. (Animal researchers have likewise observed that introducing a new partner results in increased sexual activity, a phenomenon they call the "novelty effect.")

For women without a sexual partner—or couples who want to expand their repertoire—the novelty effect may come from a "personal massager." One newspaper described as "user friendly" the Prelude 3 by Windemere, a model complete with options like the G-Spotter Plus, which allows you to work the pelvic floor muscles. Prelude 3, the newspaper quipped, offers "safe sex, reduction of wrist injuries and the joys of leaving the dweeb at the bar under the same rock where you found him."

It is possible for orgasm to be better at midlife than it was when we were younger. "During the first thirty years of married life I could arrive at orgasm through stimulation around or above the clitoris, but I couldn't tolerate direct clitoral touch," said one woman at the Yale clinic. Menopause brought her a surprise dividend. "Now I can enjoy direct clitoral stimulation and have found, for the first time ever, that I am multiorgasmic."

Some of the women I interviewed, who were in their late forties and fifties, had had prolonged periods of sexual abstinence. Not all were unhappy with the situation; some thought of it as natural, a kind of hibernation. "Five years ago I would never have imagined going several years without sex," said a 51-year-old artist. In reality, she didn't find it particularly worrisome: "I don't feel this is something that's left me and will never come back again. I mean, if you're not going to have sex, why be turned on all the time and be frustrated and unhappy? It's almost as if the body goes into a self-protective state when you don't have sexual outlets. I'm convinced that if I were to get into a relationship tomorrow, I would turn on sexually in a heart-beat."

Others told me that all it takes is the arrival of an attractive partner, and—bam—sex is on again. "I wasn't having sex at all for two years and was feeling quite desperate about it. I felt myself shrivel in a way," says Donna. "Then I met a man with whom there was a very strong connection, and I felt the return of powerful sexual feelings. I thought, 'Oh, *that's* still there?' "

The Vagina at Menopause

"I think I'm starting to shrink up a little bit," Willa reports to Catherine.

"You mean your vagina?"

"Yeah."

"You do?"

"I don't know. This guy I've been seeing is very big, so it's hard to tell."

"You may be reacting to his size."

"Yeah, whether it's dryness, or shrinkage, or whether it's his size, who knows?"

"Doesn't estrogen cream take care of vaginal atrophy?"

"It's supposed to. My neighbor Mary Pat was totally atrophied. She'd had very little sex for a long time, but then she got a new boyfriend, and that's how she found out she was . . ."

"Atrophied."

"*Totally*. And she started using the cream, and it put her back to rights."

A woman who's always seen herself as hot and sexy may experience the loss of sexual juices as a blow to the ego. A medical writer I interviewed said that when it first happened, loss of lubrication made her fear she was no longer sexually "viable." "I thought, 'Oh my god, is this going to be the end of my wonderful sex life?' "

The level of distress many women feel about this symptom is reflected in the language they use. Some of the women Ellen Cole talked to compared the way their vaginas felt to "the Sahara desert," "sandpaper," and "white parchment."

When the ovaries are pumping out an adequate supply of estrogen, vaginal lubrication generally occurs within ten to thirty seconds of arousal. But when estrogen diminishes, lubrication can take one to three minutes, and there may be less of it. Almost half the women attending a London menopause clinic complained of vaginal dryness.

Vaginal atrophy, which results from estrogen loss, is experienced by ten to twenty percent of women. The atrophy can cause infections to occur. As estrogen wanes, the cells of the vagina become less acidic and therefore less able to nourish the protective bacteria that usually live in vaginal secretions. Intercourse then irritates the vaginal walls, which leads to vaginitis. If vaginal bleeding occurs, or if intercourse becomes painful, it will dampen interest in sex—at least for the time being.

Over time the tissue between the vagina and the urethra thins, causing continence problems. Women may leak urine just before or during orgasm. Some take this in stride; others are less sanguine about it. One woman told a researcher at the Yale Menopause Clinic that her tendency to leak urine had made her phobic about having sex with her husband.

But abstaining, unfortunately, only worsens the problem. Long periods of abstinence from sex make vaginal atrophy more likely. Conversely, atrophy can be prevented, or at least diminished, by sexual activity, which stimulates the vaginal tissues, helping to prevent alterations in vaginal mucosa and secretions.

"Use it or lose it" runs the popular if ominous-sounding prescription for menopausal women. The fact is, significantly less vaginal atrophy occurs in women who are sexually active, Philip Sarrel states in *Sexual Turning Points*. Sex, whether with a partner or through masturbation, helps maintain the elasticity, and therefore the functionality, of the vaginal walls. It also stimulates lubrication. When vaginal tissue is massaged—either through masturbation or coital activity—more blood flows to the region. This causes cells to multiply and thicken, which in turn reduces atrophy. Some studies have shown that coitus plus masturbation is more effective than coitus alone in preventing loss of lubrication and vaginal atrophy.

Without enough lubrication, penetration can be painful. Vaginal lubrication normally neutralizes the alkaline ejaculate, so with less lubrication available, the ejaculate may become an irritant. Not surprisingly, women who suffer from untreated dryness are likely to experience lowered desire and may begin to avoid sexual activity altogether. If a woman or her partner thinks her slowness to lubricate means she isn't "turned on," misunderstanding and defensiveness can occur. Both partners need to know that slower, reduced lubrication is normal at midlife and is *physiological.*

Between 20 and 30 percent of women at the Yale Menopause Clinic reported a hypersensitivity that made them not want to be touched—not only sexually but in *any* way. Even their own clothing rubbing up against their bodies made them uncomfortable. "I draw back from touch now, the roughness of it. I'm afraid of being hurt," one patient told Ellen Cole.

A woman I interviewed said that while she sometimes wants sex, "other times I don't want to be touched. 'Don't come near me,' I could scream!"

It isn't known for sure what causes this aversion, but one researcher speculates that estrogen-related changes in the time it takes nerve impulses to travel from one cell to another may affect perception of touch. One 49-year-old who'd recently stopped menstruating enjoyed great sex for the first year of a new relationship. Then, gradually, she began avoiding sexual contact. "I didn't like the way it felt when he touched me," she recalls, "and we both misinterpreted what that meant. The fact that my vagina didn't lubricate anymore was sort of a confirmation."

Because neither partner understood that her lack of lubrication was normal, feelings of rejection and lowered self-esteem developed. Eventually the relationship fell apart. Sometime after the breakup, the woman began hormone replacement therapy, and lo and behold, the touch aversion disappeared. "I even went back to him recently, and the sex was like old times. But now he's pretty involved with someone else, so I guess there's no future for us. It makes me furious, actually."

ORAL estrogen returns lubrication to normal in five or six days; estrogen cream will do it even faster. Lubricants like vitamin E cream or oil, K-Y Jelly, or Replens, applied directly to the vagina, also relieve dryness (although, as earlier noted, they don't prevent atrophy).

Some women become insecure about lubricants, fearing men will be turned off by them. "I don't think I'll ever be able to get used to the mechanics of artificial lubrication," one woman told Cole. "My husband is patient and kind, but I think he's getting bored. Planned obsolescence, that's me." *Hot Flash,* a newsletter for menopausal women, suggests that the lubricant be applied by both partners during genital foreplay. "This avoids the psychological trauma of reminding the woman that her body is less responsive and that a lubricant is needed."

One woman told me she reduces the feeling that it's *her* by applying the lubricant to her husband's penis.

Hormone changes, of course, also affect sexual response in older men. Consider how the man's penis often requires certain kinds of stroking in order to become erect. Providing that stroking or kissing *could* be seen as mechanical, but usually it's just experienced as part of the natural sexual exchange. Lubricating the vagina in whatever way works can be seen, in the same way, as just another part of the sexual dance.

HORMONES AND DESIRE

HIGH levels of estrogen correlate with high levels of desire. When estrogen is low, during the two weeks before the period, most women experience a slight decline in their sex drive. Perhaps it's part of nature's scheme for perpetuating the species. Desire is greatest at the time of ovulation, which is also when estrogen spikes.

The amount of estrogen we produce—at *any* time of the

month—slowly drops as menopause approaches. This is why women may find themselves getting less turned on sexually. Midlife men begin losing *their* sex hormones, too. But in women the sex hormone drop-off is less gradual than in men, and for that reason, it can produce more noticeable effects, such as loss of desire.

Not all women become less interested in sex after menopause, but those who do may arouse little sympathy in the ones who say they never felt sexier. They sometimes exhibit a queenly attitude, as if they were just plain sexier to begin with. Or as if, through superior emotional health, they are able to ride high over the inadequacies that beset the rest of us. It's like the attitude of some women whose periods are painless toward those whose premenstrual week brings them to their knees. "It's all in their minds," the queens think.

In fact, much of it *is* in our minds—or more precisely, in our brains. Though environment certainly affects how ready, willing, and able we are for sex, brain chemistry is right up there as an influencing factor. Neuroscience has begun uncovering clues as to why desire diminishes at menopause. When estrogen drops, studies show, so does serotonin, one of the brain neurotransmitters that regulate libido. When estrogen is replaced through hormone therapy, a higher level of brain serotonin may be maintained, and with it, sexual desire.

Unfortunately, midlife women often feel guilty when their libido diminishes, and they worry about its effect on their partners. They may even accuse themselves of being neurotic. "Am I withholding from him because of something he's done earlier in the day?" a woman at the Yale Menopause Clinic asked herself. "Why have I become so petty? I never *used* to take arguments to bed."

Once we start blaming ourselves, we enter a vicious cycle: Loss of interest in sex makes us feel guilty, the guilt further diminishes our interest in sex, and so on. Not knowing that the causes of the problem are physiological and may soon disappear—not only loss of libido but insomnia and hot flashes may go away after our bodies adjust to the hormone shift—we tend to avoid what embarrasses us or causes discomfort.

A woman I interviewed who has a satisfyingly positive relationship with her second husband nevertheless worries about her vacillating desire. She is 52. "There are times when I feel very turned on and

sexual, and I really want to have sex all the time. And there are times
when I have no interest at all. That's when I get scared, and I feel,
What's wrong here? How come we're not having sex? Is there something wrong with us?"

It can be damning to compare our current levels of desire with
how we felt years ago. The woman continued, "When Richard and I
met, we were very, very sexual. So I don't know whether all that was
just part of a beginning relationship and the eros that happens, or life.
I mean, life gets in the way, it really does. I don't know if age has
anything to do with it. I don't know if there are limits I'm putting on
myself, if I'm stopping myself from really letting go. I'm not sure what
comes first."

THE diminishment of sex drive that occurs gradually as our hormone
levels drop off will be dramatically exacerbated by a hysterectomy in
which the ovaries are removed as well as the uterus.

One in two American women are told to have a hysterectomy,
and one in three do so. (In Europe, only about one in twenty-five
have this operation.) In some cases, surgery may be needed to remove
a malignant growth or other life-threatening disease, but the number
of hysterectomies far exceeds medical necessity in the United States.
One of the unfortunate results is that legions of women enter menopause prematurely. And many, if not most, haven't been fully in-
formed by their doctors about how removing their ovaries will affect
their sex lives.

"It was like one day I was me, and I was young, and the next
day—literally—I wasn't," says Delcy, describing the changes she went
through. "Overnight my sex drive was cut by three-quarters. For a
while it was cut to nothing. I mean it's chemical, goddamn it! If you
don't have estrogen, you don't have desire. You have *memories* of desire, but you do not have desire. You have *fond feelings* for a person.
You're accommodating because you love that person. But you don't
have lust."

With hormone replacement therapy, Delcy was able to regain
much of her gratifying sex life. "I'm telling you, when I had an or-

gasm, I nearly went out and celebrated. It was like, 'Oh my god, there's life!' "

VIVE LA TESTOSTERONE DIFFÉRENCE!

WOMEN have six to ten percent the testosterone men do. A third of that is produced in the ovaries. While all women lose testosterone at menopause, those whose menopause is initiated abruptly by surgical removal of their ovaries experience a sharp drop in the hormone, Barbara Sherwin reported at the 1993 Menopause Workshop sponsored by NIH. She'd wondered what effects this dramatic drop in testosterone might actually have on midlife women. To find out, she and her colleague Morrie Gelfand, M.D., administered testosterone to a group of menopausal women at the McGill University Menopause Clinic. Bingo—their desire, arousal, number of fantasies, and rates of orgasm and coitus jumped significantly, compared with women who were given only estrogen.

MENSTRUATING women, too, respond behaviorally to testosterone levels. "The menstrual cycle data show that women who have higher peak levels of [testosterone] at midcycle also report higher frequencies of sexual interest, autoerotic behavior, and sometimes coitus, throughout the cycle," Sherwin reports in a review article in *Psychobiology*. "Clearly, more work needs to be done on the role of [testosterone] in female sexuality, but the consistency in the available data pointing to its enhancing effects is compelling." In women after menopause, testosterone may be "critical" for maintaining "optimal levels of sexual functioning."

This hormone also has a pronounced effect on energy. Compared to those receiving only estrogen, Sherwin found that women with testosterone added to their hormone regimen "felt more composed, elated, and energetic." When I interviewed her at her office at McGill, she told me of a female politician who after menopause faced having to cut back her work schedule severely because of fatigue and lack of energy. Adding testosterone to her estrogen supplements restored her to the energy level she'd enjoyed before she was hit with menopause.

In Britain, giving testosterone to menopausal women to improve libido is relatively old hat. A gynecologist at Chelsea and Westminster Hospital in London prescribes testosterone pellets for about 25 percent of his postmenopausal patients, John M. Hoberman and Charles E. Yesalis reported in *Scientific American,* early in 1995.

Germaine Greer tells us, however, that in England "only women who are part of a heterosexual couple" are permitted the drug. Apparently British physicians consider testosterone so effective they fear that should single and/or gay women get their hands on it, they would wreak havoc on the empire with their postmenopausal sex. (There is a "ceiling effect" on testosterone, an upper threshold beyond which it doesn't affect sexual behavior, Sherwin says. Nor do supplements affect behavior in premenopausal women whose testosterone levels are normal.)

Greer is down on testosterone even for women who are married. "When we give a male hormone to a married woman who has lost interest in sex we are consciously tailoring her sexuality to fit her husband's; the whole business smacks of women's willingness to try anything for a quiet life," she writes in *The Change.*

The possibility that the wife might be interested in salvaging her sex life seems to escape Greer. Margaret, whom I interviewed not long after her hysterectomy and oophorectomy (see Chapter VI), was devastated when surgery took away her desire and left her, at least initially, anorgasmic. "Sex has always been a profoundly important part of my relationship with my husband," she told me. "The idea of losing that made me miserable." Taking estrogen helped her have orgasms again, but it didn't return the desire, or lust, she used to have. When I told her about Sherwin's research on testosterone, she said, "I'm talking to my gynecologist immediately."

A year later, I spoke with Margaret again and learned that her gynecologist had refused to prescribe testosterone for her. But eventually she prevailed, due to the solicitous intervention of her mother-in-law, who is in her seventies. "Darling," this woman said, "have I got something for you!"

Interestingly, Margaret had first told her mother-in-law about the usefulness of the male hormone to postmenopausal women. Her mother-in-law, who lives in Florida and is happy in a third marriage, was able to get someone to prescribe an estrogen-testosterone combo for her. "I have two bottles," she told Margaret. "Take one."

The pill combined 0.625 milligrams of estrogen—the amount Margaret had been prescribed by her own physician—and 1.25 milligrams of the magical testosterone. Two weeks after she began taking it, Margaret told me, she was having sexy dreams again and feeling renewed desire in her waking life. "Plus," she said, "the muscles in my thighs are stronger. They had begun hurting me when I went upstairs, and now I run upstairs like a girl."

Although the dose of testosterone prescribed for menopausal women is small, it has been reported to produce mild hirsutism (hair where you don't want it) in as many as 15 to 20 percent of women given it.

Unwanted hair is an emotional subject, even for some women scientists. Sheryl Sherman, the biologist who organized the NIH Menopause Workshop, told me she thinks the data are insufficient to support the theory that testosterone-produced hirsutism is reversible.

"But what you'd be doing would be replacing the amount that you had to begin with, that was lost when the ovaries stopped functioning, right?" I said.

"That's right."

"So your risk for hirsutism would be fairly low."

"Right. But don't forget that doses may vary for different people. And we don't know what that optimal dose is. And while we figure it out, women may have some unpleasant side effects."

Barbara Sherwin, who has studied testosterone use in large numbers of patients at the McGill Menopause Clinic, is more sanguine. "We use this drug a great deal," she says. "I see it in hundreds of women. There are some side effects—nothing is without side effects. But if you give a moderate dose, and we know what that is, then they're absolutely minimalized, and they don't occur in most women."

And if, heaven forfend, hair should sprout where it isn't wanted? I asked.

"We lower the dose, and it goes away," said Sherwin.

* * *

GUIDING Sherwin in determining who might be helped by testosterone is a woman's stated discomfort with her level of sexual interest—*and* the level of sexual interest she had premenopausally. "Women tell me, and this is pretty common if you ask, 'Yes, everything's great. The relationship's great. The kids are gone.' They spend more time with their husbands. They enjoy each other. But then, the women will say, 'Maybe I don't really love him because I'm simply not interested in having sex anymore.' For these women I find testosterone very effective."

If, on the other hand, the woman was never that interested in sex to begin with, Sherwin doesn't hold out much hope for improving desire with a hormone. "For those women who had a satisfying sex life before menopause, what happens to them is that they can pick up where they left off. They once again have desire. That's the difference, and it's very striking, clinically. There's no question."

Many women aren't aware that testosterone preparations are available in this country. Sherwin attributes women's lack of information to the backwardness of gynecologists—and to the taboo against lustiness in older women. "Sexuality in postmenopausal women is still not out of the closet. A lot of gynecologists simply do not ask about it because they don't want to hear about it. They don't feel terribly comfortable discussing sexuality in the first place. In the second, they don't want to elicit information if they can't do anything about it. Also, it isn't considered to be quite serious in women, or worthy of discussion. If women don't have sexual desire, they can still have sex. So it's never taken all that seriously in women, even today."

In Canada, testosterone supplements for women have been readily available for twenty-five years. One Canadian clinician I talked with, who asked not to be named because of case overload, treats high-powered professional women from the United States who are in search, chiefly, of more energy. They make the flight to Canada because they can't find anyone at home who'll prescribe testosterone. "We evaluate them and treat them in our clinic, and then do follow-up consultations on the phone."

The PC Muscles: Strengthening Our Possibilities

It's Willa, ever willing to talk about it, and Catherine, ever willing to listen.

"I'm coming faster. It seems to me that when I was younger, I could hold a certain level of pleasure—"

"Of excitation."

"Longer."

"Yes."

"It may be a muscular thing, something to do with PC muscles. Mine are a little weak, my doctor told me. Like if I jump or sneeze or anything, I pee a little."

"They say that's directly related to your sexual—"

"The orgasms, yeah. I mean, I still have great orgasms, but it's not like . . . well, they just don't go on the way they used to."

A woman who's been celibate for two years tells me she's worried because she seems to have no muscle tone in her pelvic floor. Following the advice in a sex manual, she tried, as an exercise, "cutting off the stream," but wasn't able to. "If this in fact is an accurate test, my muscles seem to have disappeared. What do I do now, just keep trying?"

After 45, most women experience some weakness of the "PC," or pubococcygeal muscles. These are the muscles that wrap around the vagina, the urinary opening, and the anal region in a figure-eight configuration, connecting to the pubic bone at the front and the coccyx at the rear. Weakness or flaccidity of the PC muscles happens naturally as a result of aging, declining sex hormones, and pregnancy.

But the condition contributes to both urinary incontinence *and* difficulty achieving orgasm. According to Winnifred Cutler, Ph.D., who does research on female sexuality at the University of Pennsylvania Medical School, the same woman who tends to leak urine may have difficulty achieving a vaginally stimulated orgasm. Weak PC muscles sometimes cause small amounts of urine to be lost during sex—especially during orgasm. This problem can be reversed, or at least greatly controlled.

The PC muscles *can* be strengthened by specific exercise. As the muscles get stronger, in three to six weeks, urine stops leaking, and clitoral stimulation more often leads to orgasm. As the muscles get stronger still, *either* vaginal or clitoral stimulation may produce orgasm. *The stronger the pelvic muscles, the more orgasmic the woman.* "If Freud and his followers had focused on helping a woman to build her PC-muscle strength rather than overcoming her childhood toilet training," Cutler suggests, "vaginal orgasms might be the birthright of every woman."

Like building up quads and pecs with a weight-training program, rebuilding the PC muscles involves repetition and doing the exercise with proper form. Dr. Arnold Kegel, who first established the connection between weak PC muscles and urinary stress incontinence, reexamined patients after they had done three to six weeks of these exercises. Much of the slack in the PC muscles had been tightened, the uterus, bladder, and perineum had assumed a higher position, and the vagina was longer and tighter. The women also reported that the strength of orgasmic contractions had increased.

The PC muscles are separate from both the stomach and the buttock muscles. When you're contracting the right set of muscles, neither the stomach nor the buttocks will tense. In fact, it isn't possible to detect from looking at you that you're doing these exercises.

To do them, you first have to locate the proper muscles (sometimes referred to as "circumvaginal"). One researcher advises, "To locate the circumvaginal muscle, sit on the toilet, spread your legs apart and begin urinating. See if you can stop and start the flow of urine without moving your legs. If you can stop and start the stream, you are using the circumvaginal muscle."

Kegel developed a biofeedback tool, a perineometer, to measure the strength of the muscles. Feedback from the perineometer can help a woman build her muscle strength faster and more substantially, according to NIH research. (To find out about renting this device, contact Leslie Talcott, R.N., 242 Old Eagle School Road, Stratford, PA 19087.)

PC exercises can be done anywhere, in a seated or standing position. When done correctly, results are virtually inevitable. Here is the regimen. Contract the muscles and hold them for as long as you can, working your way up to a count of eight to ten seconds. Then relax the muscles and repeat. Start off with fifteen contractions a day, adding ten more each week until you can do thirty-five or forty a day.

Morris Notelovitz describes another way of developing these muscles, a set of "pelvic muscle training weights." The set contains five vaginal cones that resemble tampons and range in weight from 20 to 70 grams. You start with the smallest, placing it in the vagina and holding it there for ten or fifteen minutes at a time. "You must use your circumvaginal muscle to hold the weight in the vagina—otherwise it will fall out," Dr. Notelovitz explains. "When you can hold the weight in place even as you cough or laugh, you are ready to progress to the next size."

I guess you have to be motivated. If you are, there's a toll-free number (800-328-1103) and a fee of a mere $99 for the Femina Pelvic Muscle Training Weights, manufactured by Dacomed Corporation in Minneapolis.

Sex and the Midlife Male

"All too often, discussion of changes in the sexuality of menopausal women fails to mention these most important changes in men, [even though] it is well established that sexual dysfunction in one partner can rapidly lead to sexual dysfunction in the other partner," says David Iddenden. In a study conducted at Stanford, nearly 25 percent of menopausal women said their partner "usually" had a problem with erection.

At sixty, most men are still having sex. By 68, somewhat less than three-quarters continue to have intercourse, although some who abstain are still interested, Jon Hendricks reports in *Aging in Mass Society*. By the time they reach their late seventies, only 25 percent of men are still sexually active, and they will probably engage in some form of sex for the rest of their lives.

A lessening of the frenetic sexual energy of youth, psychologists point out, can lead the way to a more conscious, relaxed, emotionally open sex life than before. *"Men can become far better lovers in their middle years,"* Maggie Scarf told a group of therapists attending a Harvard-sponsored conference on midlife couples' problems. "Their changing sexuality sets up a situation in which they are simply more vulnerable to their intimate partners."

As a man ages and his sex drive diminishes, he may need more direct genital stroking in order to become fully erect—just as a woman might need longer foreplay before she lubricates. Men who don't understand the work it now takes to achieve erection may misinterpret it as a "loss of potency," says Scarf, with old age and death not far behind.

The wife or lover of an aging man may also misinterpret his slowness to achieve erection as lack of desire, fearing that a younger, sexier partner is what he needs to get turned on. Says Scarf, "If she misconstrues what is happening, she may demand that he show his love for her—and her desirability—by being raring to go from the outset. This is a recipe for sexual disaster."

The man pressured to perform as if he were younger can develop acute sexual performance anxiety. "The lovers' bed is soon no longer a haven but the theater in which he gives his doomed and unsuccessful performance. Avoidance becomes his response. He may turn away from sex completely, or turn to someone new for validation of his desirability and manliness."

After sixty or so, a man's orgasms may feel less forceful and explosive. The refractory period—the time after orgasm before a man is able to have another—increases considerably. "The teenage male can have two orgasms per minute," says Scarf. "The male nearing sixty can have one every twenty-four to forty-eight hours."

If they don't know that these changes are normal, men can become quite distressed and assume that they're "losing it" completely.

MARILYN, a lively single woman of 62 whose first experiences with men in their fifties and sixties began when she was in her late forties, told me her lovers in their sixties all had occasional difficulties with erections—either getting them, or keeping them, or both. How she felt about this depended largely on how she felt about the man. "I happen to be secure, sexually, myself, so I never interpreted it as having to do with their feelings about me," she says. The man who was close to seventy (when she was still in her fifties) was the one with the most erection difficulty, but she loved him enough to stay in the relationship indefinitely—except that other problems intervened, she says. "He was very romantic and very loving, and I felt I could deal with the limitations of the sexual relationship."

One man never actually got hard until after he had entered her. "Somehow he managed to get himself in there even though he was limp. Once in, he'd always get an erection. He experienced a tremendous amount of pleasure from sex, and I found that exciting."

Not surprisingly, men with higher levels of testosterone tend to have more and firmer erections and more frequent sexual activity than those whose testosterone is declining. In one study, men with low testosterone were unable to form erections on command while fantasizing about sex. Given testosterone supplements, they were flooded with more sexual thoughts and greater excitement and in fact had sex more frequently.

Besides testosterone therapy, a man can boost his testosterone levels through regular sexual activity with a partner. (For unknown reasons, masturbation doesn't do a thing for testosterone levels.) Morning is generally the best time of day for midlife sex, since male testosterone levels are highest then.

Prescription drugs for high blood pressure can wreak havoc on a man's sex drive, as they can a woman's. Some men on hypertensive drugs take themselves off the medication without consulting a doctor, because they find losing their sex drive so intolerable. One college professor told a reporter for *The New York Times* that after taking the blood pressure medication, "I just went dead sexually. It was like I had been castrated. It was frightening." He stopped taking the drug, and his sexual response returned. But such drastic action is dangerous and unnecessary, since in most cases the medication or dose can be changed to alleviate the problem.

Exercise may also correct the problem. "Middle-age men who

exercise vigorously experience sexual changes that return them to the sexuality patterns of younger men as they improve their cardiovascular fitness," Winnifred Cutler reports. In one study, seventy-eight healthy but sedentary men agreed to begin jogging or biking three times weekly, and nine months later, they were engaging in sex 30 percent more frequently than before the exercise began.

Vigorous exercise is the key. In another study, 48-year-old men were divided into two groups, one group agreeing to walk three times a week for an hour, and the other agreeing to participate in a strenuous one-hour physical fitness regimen three times a week. Only the men in the rigorous program showed an increase in sexual desire and behavior.

Strenuous exercise, particularly of the aerobic kind, sets off bursts of growth hormone release. Growth hormone is the newest anti-aging star. The National Institute on Aging has spent two million dollars to explore its apparently dynamic role in keeping people young, lean, muscular, and sexy.

Vascular problems (clogged arteries, high blood pressure, and hardened vessels) are another major cause of impotence. Fully half the men who undergo coronary bypass surgery are impotent. More than a million American men are currently being treated for impotence—a fivefold increase over the last several years. One reason for the increase in treatment, according to Dr. James Baraa, a prominent urologist, is that people have finally recognized that if they want it, they can have satisfactory sex into their nineties.

How much blood rushes to the penis (causing the erection) and how *quickly,* is something that varies with age. The young adult male can become erect in three to eight seconds; an older man takes longer, and his erection subsides more easily. The muscles surrounding the blood vessels in the penis must be able to relax if those vessels are to fill up with blood. The muscles relax because they are signaled to do so by certain neurotransmitters, naturally occurring brain chemicals that send messages between nerve cells.

In 1992, neuroscientist Sol Snyder at Johns Hopkins discovered that the key neurotransmitter in this process is nitric oxide, which occurs naturally in nerves in the penis. Snyder believes insufficient nitric oxide, which is caused by too little oxygen getting to the penis, may be one of the main causes of impotence. Smoking, lack of exercise, and lack of regular sex can all affect the amount of oxygen getting to the penis. So can some of the drugs used to treat heart disease.

Other medical conditions that can cause impotence, particularly in midlife men, include diabetes, hypo- and hyperthyroidism, renal failure, chronic alcoholism, liver cirrhosis, and sickle-cell disease. Drinking more than four ounces of alcohol a day correlates with a low degree of sexual activity, according to Dr. Millicent Zacher, a reproductive surgeon who treats male infertility. Alcohol may affect the liver and its enzymes in a way that alters the blood chemistry, in turn affecting the amount of circulating testosterone.

If he's sluggish about sex, get him off the cigarettes and booze and onto a track.

The Powerful Potential of Fifties Sex

Some women express complete satisfaction with—indeed, celebrate the richness of—a long-standing monogamous relationship. "I am completely satisfied that I chose to love only my husband sexually," one reader wrote to a women's magazine. "He and I have nurtured each other sexually and thoroughly enjoy and respect each other's bodies. We've discussed our tastes and preferences and grown in our intimacy over the years. We refuse to entertain thoughts of greener pastures. We have no pie-in-the-sky thoughts about love. Love is a choice to be committed to the relationship for the long haul. When you approach it that way, you're led by your brain and not your hormones, and you become very selective."

And very secure.

Maggie Scarf reminded therapists at a Harvard-sponsored conference on couples' therapy, "If the partners can be tender with one another, and most especially treat with understanding and respect the normal sexual changes both are experiencing . . . then the sexual bond between them can be deepened and vitally enriched."

This deepening and enrichment was discussed by many of the midlife couples I interviewed. Especially gratifying was the new sexual maturity that the men expressed—their lack of interest in *Playboy* centerfolds and pretty-faced versions of what one described as "this generic woman I used to put on top of whomever I was with." Alan, 48, is involved in a two-year-old love affair with a woman of 52, the mother of three grown children. Their relationship gives him more, sexually, than he ever expected to have at this age. "I feel I understand sex a lot better and understand a little bit more what a woman is about sexually. I shouldn't say 'what a woman is about.' What's more accurate is that I feel each woman is different, and I never knew that when I was younger."

Richard, a 48-year-old therapist in his third marriage with a woman close to him in age (she is the woman quoted earlier in the chapter as worrying about their sex life being less intense than when they were lovers), is nothing less than thrilled with the new openness in their relationship. It's come on the heels of "lots of work" and a midlife epiphany for *him*. He discovered, through being challenged by his wife, that he had never been fully committed to the women in *any* of his relationships. This wife, whom he loved, basically said, "Now or never." It required a profound shift for Richard, who in some very deep way had never accepted limitations. The price, he found, had been to live a kind of half-life.

Sensuality cycles more slowly as people mature, Winnifred Cutler writes. "The urge to come and go in a heated rush should give way to a slower, more sensuous pace." Midlife women have to redo their ideas about sex not only for women at fifty, but also for men. At least some of the women in the Yale study who were having trouble with their sex lives, Ellen Cole thinks, "might have been holding an image—perhaps a male image, or a youthful image—of how sex is supposed to be." Rather than focusing on orgasm and intercourse, she says, people at midlife would do better to expand their vision of sexuality and sensuality, "a vision that might include new kinds of touch, fantasy, play, discovery."

Playing It Safe

Catherine hasn't been feeling well. Her symptoms are vague but unnervingly persistent: fatigue, what feels sometimes like a low-grade fever but isn't, and a slight sensation in the throat, as if she could get strep at any moment. The doctor says there's nothing wrong—but did he check far enough? All of us are beginning to obsess.

Richard says, "What about Lyme disease?"

Willa says she knows Bernie Siegal if Catherine wants his number.

Howard says, "What about that tryptophan you took when you weren't sleeping, in Brazil?"

Helen says, "Forget the tryptophan. What about that guy you slept with in Venice, the one you thought was a little bi?"

Catherine is feeling, powerfully, a sense of déjà vu, remembering the first time she missed her period thirty years ago, after her first experience of sex. That missed period meant pregnancy, of course. Do her symptoms, now, mean HIV? Since splitting up with her ex, she's had one lousy sexual experience, and they didn't use a condom. She tells herself the chances are one in a billion, one in a *trillion*. She tells herself it isn't *possible* for a heterosexual woman who has slept with the same man for sixteen years to strike out on her first encounter with someone else.

"Fran Lebowitz says sex is available these days if you're a kamikaze, but if you're not, forget it," says Helen.

Willa says, "What are friends for, if not to confront you about your most destructive behaviors?"

She also says you can't be too paranoid. She tells us a heart surgeon has just received a patent for a new kind of surgical glove that reduces the chance of exposure to contaminated blood. The glove is made of a thin layer of polyurethane foam sandwiched between two layers of latex. The surgeon claims the foam increases the protectiveness of the barrier without decreasing the sense of touch. Maybe, says Willa, someone should apply this sandwiching principle to condoms.

Catherine wonders how one actually goes about getting condoms. She thinks of sending away, perhaps, or of asking one of her daughters to go to the drugstore and buy them for her. Fiona tells her that in New York the drugstores deliver. Catherine reminds her that they are not in New York.

"As a woman coming to terms with her sexuality openly, loving instead of hating her body for the first time in forty-two years, I deeply resent the presence of AIDS," a reader wrote in response to a women's magazine survey. "I'm leaving a twenty-year marriage of very uninteresting sex and facing the unspeakable landscape of abstinence or possible death for exerting my new-found, hard-fought freedom."

Although initially AIDS seemed to be an issue mainly for gay men and IV drug users, it has clearly become a women's issue as well. In 1982, just 12 percent of women with AIDS had gotten it from sexual contact with an HIV-positive man. By 1986, the percentage had more than doubled.

Yet even though women are concerned about AIDS, the number who regularly use condoms and other safe-sex practices is alarmingly low. In a nationwide survey of ten thousand people, it was women and those with low incomes who were most likely to have risky sexual partners. And 71 percent of those reported *not using condoms*! "Women either don't recognize the risk, or they are not in a position where they can enforce safe-sex practices," concludes Joseph Catania, a researcher at the University of California and author of the study, which first appeared in *Science* magazine.

Norma Leslie, director of the Women's Health Education and Counseling Center at the University of Oklahoma College of Medicine, studied a group of divorced women at a large teaching hospital and found they tended to stop using birth control whenever a marriage ended—in spite of the possibility of future sexual encounters. "Could it be," asks Leslie provocatively, "that through divorce a sense of alienation occurs which causes one to feel vulnerable and detached, making sexual decision-making and planning difficult?"

Studies show that in midlife women tend to deal with contraceptives much the way they did when they were young or adolescent—in spite of the addition of the AIDS factor. If they were irresponsible then, they'll revert to that behavior later.

One of the women I interviewed, at 52, expressed the kind of equivocation about condoms typical of a girl who is ambivalent about losing her virginity. "This guy that I've been seeing—I don't know. I think he may have been out of town for the last month or something. I'll be interested to see if he ever shows up again. But we were using condoms, and then one of them broke one time, you know."

"And?"

"And so we stopped using them. It became a way of checking. He would say, 'I've been living a very celibate life,' and I would say, 'Yeah, me too.' And then we would do it without a condom. I mean, if he had said, 'I've been screwing around,' I would have insisted on condoms."

"Suppose he lied."

"Well, suppose he did. Then I'm fucked."

WHY aren't women practicing safe sex?

Some are afraid of seeming domineering or "too independent" if they insist on condoms.

Others think that leaving their brains turned on would lessen the intensity. "I'm not as fussy as I should be," says Enid. "I'll just be in the middle of it and—get carried away."

Intense, immediate experiences "can serve temporarily to strengthen one's identity and self-esteem," according to Norma Leslie. For this reason AIDS risk-taking, like sex without contraceptives, may serve as a defense against feelings of uncertain identity—just as it does in adolescence. (In the midst of a "Who am I?" crisis triggered by midlife feelings of loss, says Leslie, women may regress to behavior they exhibited when young.) To bolster self-esteem and wavering identity, the high-risk kick may be the one most likely to work— temporarily. Sex even with someone who's totally inappropriate can fill the bill.

So, in these times, can sex without contraceptives.

Althea, a New York therapist in her mid-fifties whose second marriage had just ended, found herself one evening becoming turned on to her cab driver. Somehow, the fact that he was Indian ("He had such a gentle voice") made the possibility of an encounter seem less dangerous, she told me. At the end of the ride she gave the driver her card. "He called me the next day, but I held out a month." Nevertheless, at the end of their first date she invited him home for sex.

Althea was behaving as she might have in her salad days, in the 1960s, when New York cab drivers were less pathological and AIDS nonexistent. Was she, at however great a risk, testing it?

"Is it me or is it my marriage?" some women wonder, when sex becomes more boring than David Letterman. Althea had been feeling for four years that hot sex, for her, might be a thing of the past. Sex with her husband had virtually come to a halt, and she felt juiceless and unattractive, which had a distinct effect on her identity. Hence the erotic pull she experienced in the back of a dark cab, on which she took action. It turned out her cab driver was a decent man, and she had a relationship with him for several months. Luck, you might say—but no patient of hers would have gone unchallenged for behaving in this way.

SOME women are lulled into feeling safe with someone who appears "healthy" (or as in Althea's case, "gentle"). A married woman participating in the women's magazine survey wrote that she was having an affair with a married man who "has made love only to his wife and had a single one-night stand ten years prior to our lovemaking. I am terribly afraid of being exposed to AIDS, yet I trust without reservation that this man is free of disease and healthy."

He may well be, but how often have women believed themselves "the only one," only to find out differently down the road?

Several times a week, 45-year-old Michael, a dentist, leaves his practice to rendezvous with prostitutes on his way home from work. He doesn't use condoms because he has difficulty with erections. Sometimes he snorts a line or two of cocaine to enhance the experience. His wife knows nothing about his second life and thus has no idea that she is at high risk for being exposed to the AIDS virus.

Michael's story may be more common than anyone knows. In the magazine survey, only 18 percent of the eight thousand respondents reported knowing for sure that their husbands had had at least one affair since the marriage began. Yet, revealingly, 77 percent felt at risk of getting infected with HIV! Apparently most suspected that their husbands had had affairs that remained unconfessed.

Many women are unsophisticated about the details of safe-sex practices. The HIV virus can be present even in the fluid that precedes ejaculation. Thus, to wait until intercourse to get out the condom is to wait too long. Dr. Jeffrey Pudney, one of the investigators who discovered HIV in pre-ejaculate, said condoms should be used during all stages of sex. "At the moment, most people consider safer sexual practice involves using a condom prior to ejaculation—or in the case of oral sex, withdrawing prior to ejaculation. The presence of HIV-positive cells in male pre-ejaculatory fluid means there is a risk that HIV transmission could occur during sexual foreplay." Condoms, then, should be put on before any genital contact.

Oral sex may be riskier than anyone wants to admit. Bleeding gums, cuts, and abrasions are common in the mouth. If someone with such an opening gives oral sex to an HIV-positive partner, the virus contained in pre-ejaculate, ejaculate, or vaginal secretions can easily enter the noninfected person's bloodstream.

One reason why it's so hard for people to come to terms with the dangers of oral sex is that the preventative options thus far are so unappealing. Practicing oral sex on a man who's wearing a condom, or covering a woman's vulva with a dental dam to give her oral sex, hardly conjures up images of being "transported" or "carried away," the fantasy to which so many of us still cling.

Making Choices Without Repressing Our Sexuality

A healthy response to concern about AIDS is not to repress our sexuality but to become self-loving and responsible, to exercise conscious decision-making. We can continue to embrace and celebrate our sexual selves *and* make responsible, self-caring choices—choices about who we'll sleep with, what we will and won't do during sex, and how we'll do it. But we can't wait until we're steamy with desire to think these questions through. We need to decide in advance what risks we are—and aren't—willing to take.

In a revealing magazine reader survey conducted in 1992, almost half the respondents (70 percent of the single women) said they'd changed their courtship rituals and sexual behavior because of AIDS. Nearly one in four discuss a partner's sexual history with him in depth "before even a sock hits the floor." But only 13 percent said they currently require an AIDS test before having sex with a new partner. "The best solution I've come up with," said one 56-year-old, "is for both me and my significant other to have an AIDS test, share the results, and remain monogamous for the duration of our relationship." She admits, though, that not even monogamy can be relied on.

Some women are taking precaution to the extreme. "The only safe sex," says one 45-year-old woman who went from having many lovers to celibacy, "is no sex." When survey respondents were asked, "If you suddenly found yourself single, what would you do?" 55 percent said they would "practice self-gratification" and 38 percent would "become celibate." Only 43 percent of the respondents would, meanwhile, also "look for a new partner."

Yet condoms—used consistently and correctly—greatly reduce the risk of HIV infection during intercourse. A single woman, or any woman who has even the remotest possibility of sexual contact with someone other than a no-risk partner, should always have condoms available at home and in her purse, should know how they are used, and should know how to safely remove them when sex is over.

FOR some of us, "buying protection" is the hardest part of the ordeal. "Two years of celibacy was enough for me," wrote a 47-year-old grandmother in *The Woodstock Times*. "I was free from all known sexually transmitted, life-threatening diseases. So if I was about to go all the way (I'd finally met someone who made me hope I was), I was going all the way with condoms. I took it upon myself to make the purchase."

After circling every counter in the pharmacy for over an hour, she finally planted herself in front of a rack of tiny boxes. "There were some swell pictures on a few of those boxes. Pictures of couples holding hands while peering out over the white sands and turquoise seas of the Caribbean. I dismissed those boxes immediately. I wasn't going anywhere near the water, let alone the sand. I just wanted something that would work in a clean bedroom on an ordinary bed. My serious concerns required a sedate box."

She made her choice, then waited until she was the only one left in the store. "I grabbed some candy, a Tootsie Roll lollipop—grape—and put it on the counter with the prophylactics. The woman was older than I was. She smiled at me. Obviously, this had been done before—a small innocuous purchase plus . . . But from her smile, I took it that she liked the lollipop touch. 'Strange times,' I said. She agreed."

CHAPTER VIII

MONEY OF ONE'S OWN

*Still Cinderella • Still Down at the Top •
Working Double and Nothing to Invest •
Living Like There's No Tomorrow • Old Princes Never Die •
Cold, Hard, and Uncaring: Images of Successful Women •
Getting Her Act Together • Watching What Happens to Mother •
Making It Grow • Seeing the Light*

"I JUST READ in some magazine that sex has gone down the tubes," Fiona tells Susan. "It's money now. Single women, married women, it doesn't matter. When they're fifty, or close to it, or just past it, financial security is what women are concerned about. Whereas one time it would have been sex. It would have been relationships. Even *the* relationship. It's all become secondary to finances, that's what I hear women saying."

Susan says, "I feel like if I had a few hundred thousand in the bank right now, I wouldn't have to worry about a thing. Well, maybe that's not exactly true. Maybe if I had a few hundred thousand in the bank *and* I could put this guy I'm seeing on retainer . . ."

"In our household," Willa recalls, "my father was the only one who knew about money. And it was a secret. We were never allowed to know how much he made. He was really the king of the house in terms of money. It was sort of a mystical thing, it seemed, the knowledge that he had. It wasn't knowledge to be taught, shared, and given to you to empower you. It was *his* power."

Still Cinderella

I knew what Willa meant. I had never been taught about money when I was young. I'd never given a thought to *what* my life would be. A B.A. was the be-all and end-all. After college I worked for a few years as an editorial assistant at a women's magazine. Then I married, with the "secret" of money still eluding me.

I became a writer almost inadvertently, as a way of pulling my head out of the diaper pail at a time when there were three children under the age of four crawling around our tiny New York apartment. When the kids' nap time arrived, I would force myself upright at the typewriter, propping myself with pillows to keep from slumping over. I had one hour out of twenty-four to myself, and I hoped that by keeping at it, I might be able to create something. I never imagined actually supporting myself, though—let alone through writing. A wife, in those days, wasn't supposed to even imagine it. Could I have predicted that money—how to earn it, how to spend it, how to save and invest it—would become a long-unresolved preoccupation, one that I wouldn't finally wrestle down until I was in my fifties?

As the years passed, I liked having my own writing career and dismissed its precariousness—its lack of health insurance, of a pension plan, of taxes taken out of the paycheck because there *was* no paycheck. I was paid fees, not salary. Writers consider the financial struggle of working free-lance to be the price of their independence. But at fifty, in the sleepless nights after ending my relationship, I sometimes looked back and wished I'd gone to work as a teacher like my friend Myra, who had a fat retirement coming to her at 55 and was soon going to start a new career selling beauty products derived from mud from the Dead Sea.

Myra had it made.

She also had a husband. Part of what I was experiencing had to do with being single. When I decided to leave the relationship I'd been in for sixteen years, I knew that at fifty, the probability of my hooking up with someone again was pretty low. Still, I felt prepared to go it alone. Not that I especially wanted to be alone, but I knew that I *could,* and that was important. I had a life, I had work I loved, a beautiful home, and adult children who were an enormous support and pleasure to me. And I had friends.

What I didn't have any longer was an illusion of protection, of financial backup should I need it. And I was being brought up short, as menopause arrived, by the extremely discomfiting fact that I wasn't immortal. That wonderful energy I'd always been able to tap into wasn't going to be there forever. Maybe I could keep on pumping out the work for another decade, even longer. But maybe not, who knew?

I had to face the fact that I was without a plan—emotional, financial, social, or intellectual. In my forties I'd earned a good income, but I'd spent it as if there were no tomorrow. When it came to the long haul, I'd never really thought about having to do it myself—forever. Oh my god, *forever!* On some level, in spite of the outward trappings of independence, I was still existing like Cinderella.

How easy it is to awaken at midlife with the sudden and uneasy recognition that the story line we were expecting has taken a different turn. The white picket fence has fallen, the Prince is long gone, and we are now and will continue to be responsible for our own support. There is no one to back us up when the rent comes due, no one to cover our expenses when we can't work any longer. We know this, and yet how many of us still avoid doing what we need to do to create secure futures for ourselves?

As women, we weren't raised to expect that *we* would be the ones providing the wherewithal for living reasonably comfortably, either now or in our later lives. Clinical psychologist Carol Anderson says it is essential that women get control of financial matters during these years. "Without this control, they will never fully experience their own power, self-esteem, pride and autonomy."

The decision to manage our money and invest for the future is another Choice Point for midlife women. And it's a Point on which many of us seem to waver, dangerously. Out of the sixty-five women I interviewed for this book, only two had a viable savings and investment plan and were putting an adequate amount of money away for the future!

How do we finally acknowledge that we are not doing what we

should to protect our financial futures—and then *do* it? By coming face up to this Choice Point, and learning to understand what underlies our skittishness about money and how to change our attitudes *and* our investing habits—making ourselves *secure*—we can cash in on the other rewards of this midlife transition.

Still Down at the Top

Women arrive at midlife with a huge financial handicap. "It's as though men and women are two runners setting out to run the same course," says financial writer Anita Jones-Lee, "but you put the female runner at a double disadvantage by first lining her track shoes with lead, and, to make matters worse, you give her more hurdles to jump before the finish line."

For women over fifty who work full time, the gender gap in pay widens to a chasm. Women in this group make only *64 percent* of what men their age make. Barriers may be tumbling for younger women, notes analyst Robert Lewis, but "the world of work for women over 50 reflects career choices, occupational pathways and child-bearing patterns of the 1950s."

Revisionist research tends to emphasize impressive-sounding percentage gains in women's incomes over the past ten or fifteen years, but these gains pale when you take into account the salaries they're based on. A woman who's earning $30,000 a year sees a far smaller increase, at ten percent, than the man who's earning $100,000.

We need adequate earnings if we're to have any hope of investing. In *Women and Money,* Jones-Lee notes that a woman who retires at 65 after forty years of full-time employment at the median female wage has earned, over the course of her lifetime, $818,840. Over the same period, the average male worker has earned $1,289,840. That's almost a cool half a million he has for retirement investments that she doesn't have!

Not surprisingly, men's stock portfolios are almost twice the size of women's. A Merrill Lynch study of 800 men and women between 45 and 64 showed that the mean investment portfolio for the men was $52,500; for the women it was $25,700. Not only do women have much less money to invest, they're less likely to assume the risks required for growth investments. Thus, the money they *do* have doesn't grow as much as men's.

THE "glass ceiling" is the set of invisible barriers that prevent women from moving to the top levels of their professions. Few women today make it to these levels. Extrapolating from studies published in financial journals, the best and brightest women of our generation, as they approach midlife, are likely to get siderailed before they have a chance to negotiate the pinnacle.

In 1976, *Business Week* published a story about one hundred top corporate women, the vanguard "first"—women vice-presidents, directors, and corporate partners. Ten years later it did a follow-up on those same women and found that not one held a top spot in a major public corporation—unless she had inherited the business or started her own. Most had gotten stuck in middle management. A third had left the corporate world entirely because they weren't being promoted or were being pigeonholed in public relations or personnel jobs.

From proxy statements of 800 large public companies, *Fortune* produced an even worse picture of women's chances for reaching the top. In 1990, among the 4,012 people listed as the highest-paid members of their companies, *Fortune* found *nineteen women*—"not even one-half of 1%." Pay, relative to men's, is worse than ever at the top. In the highest ranks, women make only 40 percent of what men make—even when they have equal experience.

In a study published in 1995 in *The Academy of Management Journal,* only about six percent of directors for Fortune 500 companies were found to be women. "At the current rate of increase in executive women, it will take until the year 2466—over 450 years—to reach equality with executive men," observes Eleanor Smeal, of the Feminist Majority Foundation.

* * *

In the corporate world, discrimination against women actually becomes fiercest at midlife. No matter how much expertise they may have gathered, females are kept from the upper echelons of business. You Don't Belong Here, is the clear message; You Don't Deserve What We Deserve.

The experience of Elizabeth Sobol, a Wall Street star who in twenty years rose from an entry-level analyst at a mutual fund to become a managing director and the highest-ranking woman at Kidder, Peabody, is a painful example for midlife women with ambitions of going all the way. In her peak year at the brokerage firm, Sobol earned $700,000. But at the age of 48 she felt compelled to resign because of age and sex discrimination in pay.

Sobol had experienced the antifemale bias in her field early on. In 1971, soon after starting as an analyst, she learned that the guy at the next desk, newly hired and doing the very work she was doing, was earning $2,000 a year more. Things didn't improve as the years went by; as she rose in the ranks, the gap between what she and her male peers earned only widened.

In 1981, after joining Kidder, Peabody, Sobol was made head of the firm's utility-finance department, with eighteen people under her. When she discovered that her male colleagues were making better bonuses, she felt she shouldn't complain since she was already making a six-figure salary. But the bonus discrepancies became more and more flagrant. In l987, after working on a $1.8 billion merger of two utility companies, "I got paid a $400,000 bonus, while the guy from the mergers-and-acquisitions division who worked on the deal got in excess of $1 million," she told reporter Meryl Gordon, of *Working Woman*. "I was very upset. My boss said, 'Maybe we can do better for you next year.' I should have left then."

Soon a new boss was threatening Sobol's career, even though she'd been cited as one of Kidder's most valuable employees. The new man "undermined" her completely, she says. "He wouldn't let me participate in significant decisions, and he wouldn't let me control compensation or hiring and firing."

When a superior she spoke to did nothing to rectify the situation, Sobol resigned. That was in April 1991. The firm offered her a consulting job whose terms she found insulting, and she filed suit for discrimination. A year and a half later, though, she was still unable to find work elsewhere. Headhunters told her that by suing she'd ruined her chances for getting another job.

Women take considerable risk when they lodge legal protests against bias in the workplace. The higher they've risen, the more they have to lose.

ONE reason for the "glass ceiling" is the bias, rampant in the business world, that women don't go after top-level positions because of their attachment to their families. "Because women generally still bear the primary burden of child-rearing, many well-qualified professionals who are mothers *just don't want high-pressure corporate jobs*—or decide to drop out temporarily," *Business Week* claims (my italics). The language, here, implies a male what-can-you-do? shrug: It's not *our* fault that women don't want to take on more responsibility.

In fact, due to the lack of equity in housework and child care, women who have the best earning potential pay the heaviest price. They don't get paid as much as their male peers, and they don't get to have families, either. Nearly half the women on *Business Week*'s Top Fifty list of corporate executives were unmarried or divorced, and a third who *had* married didn't have children. "I'm at the top of my profession now, and it took a tremendous amount of concentration and focus in a brief period of time," says Claudia Golden, the first woman economics professor at Harvard to get tenure. "If I were married and had kids, I probably wouldn't have had the energy."

WORKING DOUBLE AND NOTHING TO INVEST

THEORETICALLY, in marriages in which both spouses work, household chores are more equitably divided. In practice, however, they are not. Only 20 percent of the husbands of working women actually share equally in housework and child care, although their wives often believe themselves to have an equitable arrangement. When housework and child care are figured in, most employed wives work about fifteen hours more per week than their husbands—in all, a shocking *three extra months of full-time work per year*!

The final blow to women's financial security may be their greater involvement in caring for elderly parents. This extra work prevents many women from being able to have full-time jobs, according to sociologist Robyn Stone. Those who stop working altogether in order to stay home to care for their mothers seriously jeopardize their own financial futures. In the worst-case scenario, mother and daughter grow older—and poorer—together.

Women make up over 75 percent of those caring for elderly family members. To get an idea of what this costs these women, figure that at an hourly rate of ten dollars, the midlife woman who spends one hour a day on elder care is losing $3,600 worth of income-producing time each year. And many give up a lot more than an hour a day.

I'm suggesting not that women turn a cold shoulder to their elderly parents but rather that we acknowledge the costs of this responsibility and insist that it be shared—by brothers, by husbands, by government, whomever—so that we don't endanger our futures by playing the role of unpaid nanny once again.

TIME-OUT for child-rearing and elder care is part of the reason women fall so far behind financially as they grow older. Inadequate pension funding is another. Built into the system of economic discrimination against us, according to Beth B. Hess in "Aging and Old Women: The Hidden Agenda" is the fact that pensions belong almost exclusively to the "core" economic sector—that is, white men—and do not extend to the "peripheral economic sector," which of course includes women. Eighty percent of all retirement-age women have no private pension plan, and those who do have one get less, since pension funds are based on earnings. The average annual pension for men, a recent study shows, is $9,460. *Less than half that*—$4,330—is what women get.

Often it isn't until midlife that women begin to see that they've been doubly penalized. As a result of having been exploited earlier in their working lives, they suffer greater financial insecurity later. Those who left work to raise a family may have long gaps without salaries that will pinch back their Social Security benefits. Women's lifetime earnings are only two-thirds of men's, and their Social Security benefits reflect that. Annually they receive $4,226 in benefits compared with men's average benefits of $7,342. Should a woman have nothing else to live on, that's a pretty terrifying figure. Imagine spending the last twenty-two inflation-ridden years of your life with nothing but the current average Social Security payment for women: $608 a month!

The later years of women's lives show pitiably the effects of life-long discrimination. Over the age of 65, twice as many women as men—or 2.5 million—live below the poverty threshold. And their poverty, as they get older, increases. Almost half of older women have median incomes of less than $5,000 (as compared with one in five men). In 1990, women accounted for nearly three-quarters of the elderly poor.

LIVING LIKE THERE'S NO TOMORROW

UNDOUBTEDLY the cards are stacked against us. Women are still working twice as hard as men and earning less money. They are still being exploited as the unpaid child- and elder-care workers of the nation. But perhaps most insidiously, they are economically endangered by their own ambivalence, rooted in an unconscious wish to be taken care of.

Rhoda, who lives in Chicago and thinks of herself as having always been independent (she is three times divorced and has supported herself for years), says, "I certainly can't count on some guy being there to support me, and I don't want to be dependent on my children. So I feel like I really have to get some money together for retirement."

But then again, she thinks, maybe it isn't really necessary. "Who knows," she says, switching tracks. "Maybe I'll just keep on working. Maybe I'll *always* be able to work."

The fantasy of immortality is more comforting than facing the inevitability of age and the need to prepare for it.

RHODA has a small business that provides word-processing and other services to writers. She keeps mornings for herself, however, and each day sits down diligently at her computer, learning how to write a screenplay. She figures that even though it may take her five or ten years to learn the craft, she could make a killing if she ever actually sells a script. "Think of what writers get on just one film!"

She's enjoying the full scope of her creative powers for the first time in her life, but she's also gambling three hours of her precious time each day—fifteen hours a week. In the meantime things are tight, so tight she has decided to cancel her medical insurance. "I'd rather take that $150 a month and put it into an IRA or a Keogh than—well, I guess it's a gamble at this point."

"Suppose you become sick?" I say.

"Well," she says, "if I became sick . . ." She doesn't finish the sentence but shifts to a more comforting idea. History is on her side. "I haven't been sick since 1969," she says. "Literally. *Nothing.*"

"But statistically," I persist, "the chances of something happening to you are much greater with every passing year."

"Yeah, but before giving up my medical insurance, I had everything checked—*everything.*"

"And you have a clean bill of health."

"I have a totally clean bill of health. And also, I'm very tuned in to my body, so I think that if anything ever started—"

"What would happen if anything . . . started?"

"Well, I would *know* it, you know what I mean?"

As the women's movement got into swing in the 1960s and 1970s and women began making money for the first time, we also began spending it—with abandon. After finally achieving financial independence, and sometimes at great cost, we didn't want limits placed on our ability to spend. No one was going to tell *us* we couldn't spend $200 on a pair of Joan and David shoes or $2,000 on a ski week in Zermatt.

But women in our age group reveal a surprising lack of financial savvy. Half between the ages of 35 and 54 have checking accounts that pay no interest. Only 12.5 percent own stock or mutual funds, and only 6 percent have money market funds. Those who actually manage to invest don't begin doing so until midlife. The average female stockholder is 49, compared with the average male stockholder, who is 44.

Even women who earn a substantial income often have a hard time making the commitment to save and invest money. Says a successful photographer, "Whenever I've made big chunks from a royalty or foreign sale, the accountant will tell me, 'You really should put money into your retirement account.' So begrudgingly, I'll put something in. But if he weren't there guilt-tripping me, I'd spend everything I make. As it is, I haven't put away nearly enough."

Divorced women often spend their divorce settlements on luxuries, perhaps in an effort to compensate for whatever they had to put up with in the marriage—or for the trials of leaving it. Widows, too, spend, and spend fast. Eighty percent of widowed women zip through their insurance settlements within eighteen months of receiving them. Some lose the money in unsound investments, one study shows; others simply blow it.

It goes against the grain tremendously to siphon money away from the present and put it aside for the "future." I still believe no one would do it who wasn't trained to do it, as seals are trained to jump for fish. But middle-class males are so trained. Beginning at their father's knee, they are taught to plan and scrimp and save so as to be able to grab on to and maintain a certain standard of living. Not so middle-class females. We grew up expecting to be swept off to a retirement condo in West Palm, just as, in our twenties, we imagined we'd be swept off to the white cottage with the picket fence. This dream of being swept away is not something we choose, but we harbor it nonetheless. It's what *we* learned at our mother's knee, and although we have attained a certain amount of independence, the dream of rescue lingers on. It's what we mean when we think, however anxiously, "the future will take care of itself."

Most of us never really imagined we would have to take care of ourselves up until the very end. "*I* can do this," we thought, as the women's movement swept us forward in the 1970s. But we may also have secretly believed, "I won't have to do this *forever*." When it finally dawns that there's no one but *us* to support the last several decades of our lives, we may not have invested one cent. It's the Cinderella Complex revisited, only now there's little time left in which to make up the shortfall.

Old Princes Never Die

Some women equivocate on the issue of self-support even when they've been earning their own income for years. Nor does the amount of money they earn have much bearing on the matter.

"I don't think I'm ever going to retire. I don't *want* to retire," insists Maryanne, a medical writer. At least she invests, plunking chunks of money into a Keogh account that an old college friend manages for her. And she is proud of her success—understandably. She hopes it will go on forever. "Seeing what people look like at sixty-five, I would think I have at least fifteen more good years working at the pace I'm working now. Then, if I had to, I could slow down."

Has she put together a big enough cushion to be able to do that? "I don't spend a lot of time thinking about it," she says. "Maybe I'll buy a house with a little cottage on the property that could be an income unit. Also, probably David and I—I'm looking forward to being together with him. And two people can live, you know—"

"Cheaper than one."

"Right. We'd both be bringing in some money."

Maryanne seemed to veer back and forth between feeling powerful enough to work forever and experiencing the terror of mortality. "The only thing I'm afraid of," she told me, "is illness and death. Getting cancer is terrifying to me. Getting some awful thing like breast cancer. You know, one day you wake up and you've got breast cancer, and it's in your lymph nodes. Or you break a leg. I don't know. You lose your eyesight in a car accident. Those kinds of natural disasters."

Life is a crapshoot, in other words. We're not really in control. And as for success, isn't it really tempting fate? "Sometimes I think I'm so happy and everything's so good that something bad is going to happen to me," Maryanne concludes. "Something terrible."

Death by cancer and utter destitution remain the crippling fears of many women at midlife. God forbid we should be successful, happy, and secure, having prepared solid futures for ourselves. To earn money, invest smartly, and create new money is brazen, risky. It flies against everything we've been taught is womanly—and safe.

WHILE attending a conference in New Orleans, I met a lovely woman from Baton Rouge. Serena has a full-time practice as a Jungian psychotherapist, a grown daughter, and a husband to whom she's been married for thirty years. At 51, she found herself beginning to look anew at the "security" she'd known all her life—the house, the land, the horses. She was having strange dreams, she told me. A change seemed to be in the offing. She didn't know what sort of change, she just felt she was on the verge of something. I asked if I could interview her, and she agreed.

Serena, dressed simply in flats and Eileen Fisher linens, is one of those southern women who in her quiet, refined way gets what she wants. We met in her hotel room, which I immediately noticed was twice the size of mine. How had she managed that? Sweetly, she said, "I didn't like the room they gave me, so I asked what was the best room they could possibly give me without my having to pay anything additional."

The setting sun loomed large in the west window. Books, mostly of a spiritual bent, were stacked neatly on her coffee table. A journal in which she writes each day lay there as well. During the two-day conference Serena took most meals in her room so that she could read while she ate—in all, a serious woman, a thoughtful woman. And apparently, a *secure* woman. But that was only surface. "Every now and then," she told me after we'd talked for a while, "I get an icy chill. I think I'm going to die in poverty. Or I'm going to wind up without a penny and at the mercy of someone, or the system."

Although she earns her own income, Serena somehow doesn't look upon it as *hers*. Like many women, she lets her money drift into the family pot without thinking much about her own future. "I've totally relied on our life together as my retirement," she told me. "The only thing I have on my own is an IRA. I put two thousand dollars into it every year at tax time."

"Do you invest that money?"

"My husband does. It's his field. He's in finance."

As difficult as it is for many women to accept, men don't always make investments with their wives' best interests in mind. Sometimes their decisions have the effect of maintaining their wives' dependency on them.

At 52, Barbara plans to retire from teaching in two years. Soft-spoken, with a wry sense of humor, she's married to a school principal who controls the couple's money. This wasn't always the case. "Ron never even used to balance my checkbook; he'd just put a hunk of money into it every month. But the year I turned fifty, I began talking about the possibility of us splitting up."

When Barbara began to talk of divorce, a light went on for Ron. "He suddenly realized that with my name on everything, along with his, I had access to all of the money. Immediately he switched every last account into his name. Even my car, which I make payments on, is in his name now. He figures if I'm going to go, it'll be with nothing."

"You mean if you want to write a check, your husband has to sign it?" I said.

"Yes," she admitted.

"How does that feel?"

"Well," she said, "somewhat uncomfortable. But my girlfriends have much less money than I do. The economy is so bad, people just don't have much money to spend. It's been pretty easy for me to adjust. The friends I used to go to New York with shopping, they just *can't,* now, for various reasons. . . ."

"But do you have any feelings about the fact that *he's* the one who's doling it out?" I tried to return the discussion to her.

"Yeah, it annoys me. It does annoy me."

"But you put up with it."

"I don't live so badly," she says.

Women whose husbands control the money often like to imagine they'd handle it better if they controlled it. It's like backseat driving:

You get the glory of being the better driver but you don't have to take the risks involved in actually doing the driving. Serena told me she's always been the more responsible one, steadier, more cautious about spending. Her financial-wizard husband used to run up the credit card bills, which got them into trouble until she put a stop to it.

"But you still allow the money to remain in his hands," I noted.

"Yes," she said, then offered a psychological explanation. "In Jungian terms a person really can't grow up until they get rid of, or integrate, the 'daughterly attitude.' The daughterly attitude is, 'Someone will take care of me. Someone will ultimately tell me how to lead my life.' "

Serena is struggling with that. "What has happened here? Why am I not in charge of my own retirement?" she asks herself. It puzzles her that she is still so passive.

"How do you imagine your husband would react if you were to tell him you wanted to deal differently with your finances?"

"Probably he'd be very upset. It would interfere with his style, that's for sure."

"Meaning?"

"Meaning his freedom to use our collective money for anything he wants, which is pretty much the way it's always been."

Serena's husband not only has complete access to her money, he virtually owns it, since Louisiana is still on the Napoleonic Code. "It requires a great deal for a woman in this state to become totally and a hundred percent participating in the family's money. It has to be accomplished by a legal act, and then the man loses his sole rights over the family money, which is what Ron now has."

Independence is relative. It's a matter, as they say, of where you're coming from. That Serena has a personal checking account and her own IRA may make her as revolutionary in Baton Rouge as some feminist activist in the north.

"WOMEN who divorce generally end up with less money, less earning potential, and less likelihood of finding a new partner," says noted family therapist Monica McGoldrick. Divorce, for most women, brings financial disaster. Virtually overnight they can take the plunge from an upper-middle-class lifestyle to near-poverty. A California study found that in the first year after a divorce, men's standard of living went up 42 percent while women's deteriorated 73 percent.

Once the marriage is over, most women never catch up with their former standard of living. Ten years after divorce, 80 percent of the men in one study were financially secure or very secure, compared with 20 percent of the women. By the time they're of retirement age, *over one-third of divorced women are poor or near-poor.* If they haven't logged enough salaried quarters, they may not be eligible for Social Security benefits *or* a pension.

Most women who are divorcing don't ask for alimony, saying they want to be "free and clear" of their ex-husbands. They may blame themselves for the failure of the marriage and feel guilty about asking for money—even in cases where they were a partner in launching the husband's career. "Regularly in my practice," says Dr. Martha Kirkpatrick, "no matter what the marriage experience has been, no matter how fearful the expectations of punishment, no matter who initiates the divorce or why, the woman begins by announcing she is lucky that her husband is an honest and responsible provider and will not cheat his family of adequate support."

Thus does the Prince-fantasy linger on, solacing the unwitting Princess with the illusion of patriarchal protection. The divorcing women who come to Kirkpatrick for counseling still view their husbands as the Great Provider, although, she says, "evidence of this husbandly trait is often not forthcoming."

Spousal support is awarded in less than 14 percent of all divorces, and it is received in less than 7 percent. Almost one in five men who have been ordered to pay alimony fall behind in their payments within six months of the divorce. Moreover, although property is said to be settled equally these days under no-fault laws, only the tangible assets are covered. Career assets, such as salary, pension, medical insurance, education, and future earning power generally stay with the husband, Kirkpatrick points out.

In addition, women with children *usually* end up supporting them. Only 20 percent of divorced fathers are in full compliance with their child-support orders, and only another 15 percent partially comply. Whether they are single, divorced, or widowed, *most* mothers—59 percent—end up being the *sole* support of their children!

Women who never marry at all may end up better off than widows and divorcees—they retire earlier and, more often, with a pension—although they're still less likely than men to save or invest. Even at midlife, social scientists have noted, a single woman may harbor the fantasy that one day someone will come along to provide for her. Thus, taking measures to create permanent income and an adequate retirement fund would mean acknowledging the likelihood that the Prince isn't coming. By the time she finally gets around to this, she may have lost years of saving and investing.

COLD, HARD, AND UNCARING: IMAGES OF SUCCESSFUL WOMEN

BECAUSE success in the marketplace is attributed to ruthlessness and competitiveness, women at the top are often viewed as "not typically feminine, and singled out for attention that is not altogether flattering," write Annette Lieberman and Vicki Lindner in *Unbalanced Accounts: Why Women Are Still Afraid of Money*. In one study the authors asked women to imagine themselves at a chic dinner party seated next to a successful woman who was earning a lot of money in their same field. The women were asked to describe that dynamo—how she looked, what kinds of feelings she brought up.

Cold, severe, hard, forbidding, unpleasant, unfeminine, even "evil" was what women had to say about the Successful One. "She's wearing black and pearls," a video writer imagined. "Extremely plain and kind of severe, with a thin, slightly drawn face. I can't relate to her at all. She feels that I'm some underling that might want something from her that she doesn't want to give. I'm very reserved."

Unconsciously, some women fear that economic independence will transform them into cold, "unfeminine" creatures who will be rejected by men and shunned by other women—who, in essence, will find themselves alone at the top of the iceberg. The predicament of these women is heightened at midlife, for lying right on the other side of the Bitch in Pearls image they hold of the successful woman is the phantom Bag Lady, with her plastic dry cleaning bags and rickety shopping cart. It is the specter of destitution that haunts us in the middle of the night.

Fear of ending up destitute is a preoccupation of one in two educated, middle-class women, surveys have found. That fear, I think, has to do with the complicated relationship women in their fifties and sixties have with money. You need training and encouragement to feel capable of lifelong self-support, and we were late in getting that.

When Allison, who lives in Fairfield, Connecticut, got divorced, like many women of her generation she believed that it was wrong to ask for alimony, even though she'd spent her prime working years rearing five children while her husband launched a successful business. In the divorce settlement she got enough money for a down payment on a house, and that was it. At 47, she began a new career in teaching. Today, at 67, she's three years away from qualifying for a pension. "But I'm scared to death," she says, "because the income I'll get is small. And since I didn't work outside the home all those years, my Social Security payments will be low, too. Lately, I've been having thoughts about ending up a bag lady."

This fear, so prevalent among women, is not entirely unfounded. One in five older women *do* live in poverty. Still, the image of the Bag Lady has become the symbol for a variety of vague, ill-confronted anxieties particular to our generation. Of course we fear the isolation and powerlessness associated with being old. But more than anything we may be panicked about our own passivity—our resistance to creating true security for ourselves. "I'll be out on the street and I'll die— alone and lonely," Allison continues. "And it's not the poverty I fear so much as not having a home that I can control."

A home to control is the bottom line for women who fear they aren't going to be able to make it in the world. What would Allison do if she were to end up "out on the street"? How would she defend herself against the elements?

Don't think she hasn't thought about it. "I'd make a house out of cardboard," she says, "just like the bag ladies do."

*   *   *

CONTRARY to women's fear that earning power and competence with money will make them unattractive to men, those Lieberman and Lindner have studied who were "good" with money also tend to have good relationships. "Modern women who enjoy sex as well as money have a strong sense of self-esteem, freedom, and control over their destinies," they write. "They are successful sexually for the same reason that they're on top of things financially—because they've taken responsibility for themselves." Women who reject the idea of financial success, the researchers found, were the ones most likely to be without men, or to be in troubled marriages and love affairs.

At midlife, we have the opportunity to forge new identities as money-competent women.

GETTING HER ACT TOGETHER

RECENTLY I listened to an old tape of *I'm Getting My Act Together and Taking It On the Road*, that 1970s musical by Gretchen Cryer and Nancy Ford that took women by storm. Rooted in Gretchen's own experience, the play dramatized resoundingly the struggle and the exhilaration women of our generation experienced as we worked our way free of the traditional roles imposed on us.

Almost twenty years ago, I interviewed Gretchen on the heels of her success, and I wondered now what had happened to her in the interim. What kind of woman-in-her-fifties had she become? I called her, and she invited me to come to her Manhattan apartment and talk.

When I arrived at her building, several blocks from where I had lived when my kids were growing up, Gretchen was waiting for me at the front door. "You look exactly the same!" we both shrieked.

She was still the same size six, her hair was still long and dark and curly. She has deeply smiling eyes and a great wide smile. It was hard to believe, but Gretchen was a grandmother. Her recently divorced daughter is living with her, along with her four-year-old granddaughter. "I know they won't be here forever, but right now it's great," says Gretchen.

Gretchen grew up in the 1950s, and her story is like that of many of us. In those years a woman's expectations were riding on college—where you were expected to get pinned, engaged, and then married to a doctor, lawyer, or minister.

In 1957, Gretchen graduated from college and married Don Cryer, who was headed for divinity school and a life in the ministry. "While he was being the Minister, I would be the Wife of the Minister," Gretchen told me, mimicking her girlhood dream. "I imagined having a little drama group for the high school kids in the church basement."

Of course it didn't work out that way. Early in the marriage, Gretchen's husband left the ministry to become an actor. She followed him to New York and eventually started work in the theater herself. Gretchen did some songwriting in those years, but mostly she took care of the kids and backed her man through the lean years of his career. Then, after eleven years of marriage, he fell in love with someone else.

She was 33 then and overnight a single mother. "I had to leave behind all those patterns and expectations and forge a new existence for myself." Still, there was a payoff for Gretchen. Don Cryer's falling in love with someone else, she says, became a catalyst. "I kept thinking, I want to *write* about the journey a woman like me had taken from that 1950s sensibility, totally buying the program, accepting this whole set of expectations and being the 'good girl,' and then divorcing and having to redefine my life in totally new terms. I kept thinking, 'I want to *write* about that.' "

One night, while she was singing in a club with her writing partner, Nancy Ford, it came to her. "I'll write a play about a cabaret singer who's writing a whole new act for herself. That will be the metaphor for the new life she's creating. She'll call it, *I'm Getting My Act Together and Taking It On the Road*."

Joseph Papp, then the director of the American Shakespeare Festival Theater, produced the show and it became a long-running hit.

Gretchen hadn't expected to perform in it as well, but Papp wanted her to. So she opened her throat and strutted into a new career.

Twelve years, then fifteen years went by, and Gretchen's life changed. "I've always had this incredible sense that I could do anything, and of course that was totally false. But until I reached fifty, I had never run into the brick wall of my limitations. It started, actually, when I was forty-eight, when, in spite of my best efforts, I was unable to help my brother, who was diagnosed with a brain tumor. I had had the illusion that I could save him. I'd always been the one in the family that could save every situation. If it were a financial need or a physical need, or if someone's house needed painting, I would take care of it. But suddenly my brother got ill. I tried with all superhuman effort to help him, and he died anyway."

He lived for only three months after his cancer was first diagnosed. For Gretchen, that small window of time changed everything. "I absolutely, on a gut level, had to face my limitations."

Not long after her brother died, her parents "went down," Gretchen says. It was a doubly tragic day. Her father, who six weeks earlier had suffered a paralyzing stroke, slipped and fell while getting out of bed. When her mother tried to pull him up, three of her vertebrae collapsed.

Having begun work on a new play about Eleanor Roosevelt, Gretchen suddenly had to start commuting to Indiana to take care of them. Every two months or so she'd go out and spend a few weeks, trying to get the house renovated so that her father could move around it in his electric motor scooter. "I'd cook like mad for them, then come home, do a little bit of work, and soon be flying back out there again."

Inevitably, the expense and the stress became too much, and Gretchen had to devise another solution. She began preparing her parents' meals at home, packing them in dry ice, and FedExing the box to Indiana. "Every two weeks a package would arrive, and they would withdraw layer after layer of cooked meals and baked goods and put it in their freezer. It provided such a lift to their spirits, it was transforming."

Her parents loved the arrangement. Soon her mother suggested to Gretchen that she start a business. "It hit me the same way an idea for a musical hits me. I thought, 'There's such a *need* for this, for women in midlife who've just gotten their kids out of the house and now their parents go down flat.'"

"The Extended Family," the new business was called. Gretchen knew she had made a life-changing decision. "I, who had shied away from business my whole life, not even wanting to do my taxes, was suddenly going to have to raise the money, make a business plan, go convince bankers, find someone who would operate the plant. Even brainwise, it was a whole different kind of activity."

Where does the motivation for making such change come from? For Gretchen, it came from confronting the reality of her second half—the recognition that she had to support herself in this new stage of adulthood if she wanted to enjoy it.

What had happened to her parents was woefully instructive. "Because they had no money, my son and I had to bail them out. They hadn't laid aside a thing, *nothing,* not twenty dollars."

Suddenly Gretchen saw the reality of her career in show business in a new way. "You can have some very good years, as I did after *Getting My Act Together,* but then there are years when nothing comes in. I thought, 'My god, in twenty-five years, when I'm their age, am I going to be in the very same position, without a penny, and having to rely on my kids to support me?'"

Starting this business, she says, was a way of looking at her future and saying, "Maybe I can set up something that twenty years down the line will yield what I need to live."

She went after her idea big time, persuading her partner's father, William Dumke, CEO of Henningsen Foods, to share his knowledge of the food business and help her secure loans—a half-million dollars from a savings bank and another $150,000 from the Small Business Administration. Private investors contributed an additional $200,000, and Gretchen was in business. She hired a woman to run the plant while she remained in New York City, marketing The Extended Family from her office at home. She was the owner and founder of a business that had never before existed.

Gretchen hadn't gone to school to learn how. "See that basket?"

she says, pointing to a Brazilian beauty as high as the side of my chair. "It's filled with *Inc.* magazines and copies of *Executive Woman.* I read constantly. It's how I teach myself how to do this."

Ten months after starting the business, Gretchen had to expand drastically, tripling her freezer space. Today, with a staff of thirteen, her business mails out almost two thousand meals a week.

Thus far, The Extended Family has been financially draining for Gretchen. "I put money into it to start. I haven't taken a salary, and I've had to take out a second mortgage on the house I bought with the money from *Getting My Act Together.*" At present, she's mortgaged to the hilt. "If this business fails, I'm wiped out. I'll have nothing."

This is the sort of risk males take at midlife. Now, women, too, are jumping in, attempting to raise the ante for themselves as they prepare for the decades ahead.

WATCHING WHAT HAPPENS TO MOTHER

I knew my own view of the future had undergone a change when I started to feel differently about the place where my mother lives. A retirement community, Sandpiper Village had always seemed to me a waiting-to-die community. In some sense, it is. Still, I was amazed that on a college teacher's salary, my father had been able to organize things so that when the time came, he and my mother were able to go to this place with a swimming pool and flowered wallpaper in the dining room. How had he managed this? I wondered. He had never mentioned it, and I had never asked. But when they were old, my parents were able to live in a place where people served meals so my mother didn't have to. A place with someone to clean and look after the lawn. A place where, when the need arose, a nurse was available to drive the beleaguered inhabitants of Sandpiper Village down Route 17 to the next set of traffic lights, then over to the hospital.

When they first left their comfortable brick home in Columbia and moved into the little two-bedroom apartment in a gray wooden building connected to other gray wooden buildings by a covered walkway, I was depressed by what I saw as their reduced circumstances. But now that my mother is alone (and, of course, I see myself in her), I have a different attitude. When I think of Sandpiper Village I say, thank God. Thank God she has her friends, her meals prepared for her, her quiet carpeted abode with the little music studio and her piano and recorders and tambourine. Will I have such security when I'm her age?

The truth is, even so, that my mother has concerns about money. She and my father didn't expect to last so long. He certainly never expected that, with her sicknesses, she would live deep into her eighties, while he would be felled in a single swoop by a dilapidated furniture van on the service road by Kentucky Fried Chicken. He didn't think of this possibility, even though he'd spent his life trying to imagine every conceivable one.

After my father died, my mother's Social Security payments got knocked almost in half. Thirty thousand dollars out of her nest egg were sucked away in a matter of weeks by the company that provided the private nursing he'd needed. I was shocked by how little she'd ended up with. Yet the money my mother was left with is more than what I have put aside for retirement, even though I have already earned a great deal more money, at this point, than my parents ever did. I don't foresee ending up with as much money for retirement as they did, unless—and this strikes me painfully, as in a bad dream—I change my ways.

Today my mother's money, still in the CDs in which she so proudly—and successfully—began investing in the late 1970s, is no longer productive, but she doesn't know how to invest in anything else and would probably consider it too risky anyway. At 86, staying ahead of inflation is the farthest thing from her mind. She has other things to stay ahead of. Still, her financial situation is precarious. It saddens me that she has this to worry about, on top of everything else.

It costs my mother a little over thirteen hundred dollars a month to live at Sandpiper Village. That includes two meals a day. It doesn't include her electricity and telephone expenses, her clothing, her gas, or anything else. My mother marshals her Social Security income and her few remaining annuities with strictness and vigor, checks her medical bills to be sure she isn't being overcharged, buys an occasional skirt from L.L. Bean, and is long overdue for some new sheets. "I have enough money for another two years," she'll say. I tell her, Don't worry. I tell her I'll take care of her when the time comes. And I will, somehow.

As we watch what happens to our mothers, we are brought up short, for in their lives, now, we see our own futures. It can become a powerful impetus to change. My mother is fierce about doing what she was taught to do to protect herself in old age: She is vigilant about spending and conservative in investing. But she didn't imagine living as long as she has. In any event, her reality—the reality of her generation of women—is different from ours. We *know* the chances are good that we'll live into our eighties. And for us, the rules have changed. We'll be left with no nest egg, masterfully and silently planned for us by our husbands. What future security we enjoy will be what we have created, whether or not we have husbands. And as society's rules change, so must our images of ourselves. We cannot afford to cling to some outmoded notion of "femininity" if that's what's standing in the way of our behaving actively and aggressively to protect our futures.

Making It Grow

"Hey," says Willa, looking at a *Time* magazine report on the notorious Whitewater investment scheme, "if Hillary can do this . . ."

Catherine says, "I used to thumb through *Money* magazine on an airplane and see that some chipper young nurse had started investing $2.50 a week in a mutual fund at the age of thirty-five, and now, at forty-two-and-a-half, she's a millionaire. It made me feel inept and over the hill."

"Stories like that used to make me rue the fact that I didn't begin saving forty years ago," says Willa, "but I've recognized there's a lot I can still do to take care of myself."

One of the first rules of investing is to start early. For the Mamas, the first rule is to *start,* period. "Consider this," says Willa, clicking on Managing Your Money in her computer directory. "If a woman invests five thousand dollars a year at an average annual yield of ten percent and pays thirty-five percent in taxes on the interest, assuming a five percent inflation rate, at the end of ten years she will have the tidy sum of $78,057. Ten years. I mean, *we* can do ten years. We can do twenty years."

FOR some women, divorce is a call to action. "When I left my husband ten years ago I was making nineteen thousand dollars a year," Maryanne recalls. "And this was doing the same work I'm doing right now, although of course I've branched out." Now, she's making $100,000. "Every year my income keeps going up, exponentially. But I don't spend; I spend very little."

"So what do you do with the extra money?" I ask.

"I save it. I invest in mutual funds and tax-free municipal bonds. Because I'm in a medical field, I believe biotechnology is the wave of the future, and I've invested money in that. I also invest in the health care sector, because I think that's very stable."

Maryanne has become more confident as her investments began paying off. She used common sense and didn't put all her money with one broker. And she's also made money on her own, without a broker, investing in a mutual fund. "You can call a toll-free number, ask questions about what you're interested in, and make your investment," she said, marveling at the independence possible.

Women used to be taught that "preserving principal" was the cleverest financial strategy they could hope to pull off. Don't take chances, don't live off your capital—if you were lucky enough to have been left any capital in the first place. The idea was that we couldn't be expected to figure out how money works, much less be creative enough to make it grow.

While earning more and spending less is crucial for protecting financial futures, today, investing is equally important. Financial counselors advise learning to live on 90 percent of whatever you bring home and socking the other 10 percent away. By this they don't mean putting ten percent in a savings account, they mean investing it. It's through investing that men make real money.

Women tend to be excessively conservative, analysts say, keeping too much of their money liquid, available, and nonproductive. One reason women fear the risks involved in high-return investments such as stocks is that they're caretakers. They want to keep savings available in case they're needed for the household. Surveys show that women are more likely to save for their children's education, a home, or a car, while men are more likely to save for retirement.

Growth investments involving some risk are necessary if we're going to create enough money to protect our futures, today's analysts say. Psychologically, that may mean being able to tolerate anxiety— the anxiety involved both in giving up the money to the investment and in being able to ride out market volatility. Today, being financially responsible means being aggressive. We can't just be good girls, paying our bills on time. Surveys show that women are more cautious than men, probably too much so, *The New York Times* reports. "They tend to put less of their money in stocks, the riskiest but best performing investment over the long run."

If we want to build security, we have to use our money to create more money; we have to make it grow. This involves calculated risk-taking. And it involves educating ourselves sufficiently to be able to make those calculations.

In a kind of public relations experiment, Merrill Lynch brought together a group of three dozen women who had money but were afraid to invest it. "No matter what I do with money, I feel I'm doing something wrong," said a sixty-year-old vice-president of a chemical company. It soon became clear, as the seminar progressed, that she was speaking for most of the other women. Their main obstacle to financial success was fear. One woman had kept all her money in a savings account that yielded a pittance, and she owed more on her credit cards than she'd saved; her goal, she said, was "not to have to worry." But she didn't believe she could learn to handle money, and apprehension stalked her.

Overcoming fear of poverty emerged as one of the central themes of the Merrill Lynch seminars. As the seminar weeks went by, it became apparent that the women were paralyzed by ambivalence. When asked to explore the meaning money held for them, many spoke poignantly of "freedom" and "independence," as if these were states that would forever elude them.

But why were these teachers, corporate executives, entrepreneurs, and other professionals able to act independently in their work lives but not on their own behalf? During the seminars they began to see that they had backed off from taking responsibility because it meant, as one woman put it, "giving up the fantasy that someone is going to come along and take care of me." Girding herself, she added, "I'm fifty, now. I'm in the second half. It's time."

A deep feeling of second-class citizenship, of lack of entitlement that may go back to our earliest conditioning, can stand in the way of our being financially active. Gay-Darlene Bidart, a widowed painter and writer for whom money had long been "a moral puzzle"—meaning she had never felt she deserved it and she didn't know why—learned, finally, to stop feeling guilty about her money. Apparently Merrill Lynch had not been above creating a kind of tent meeting, revivalist atmosphere in order to get these women over their fears of investing. Bidart recalled, "Women were invited to come up to the front of the room and claim what was theirs: the right to learn, the right to have, empowerment. Don't hold back, we were told."

Whatever it takes. By the end of four meetings, these women had gotten the message: Ambivalence is dangerous. Greater affluence is a perfectly reasonable goal, and a knowledge of sound investing is available for the asking.

Seeing the Light

Fiona has this idea that some women like living on the edge. She says they thrive on a certain amount of just-manageable chaos. It keeps them feeling, underneath, as if they were in need of rescue. It keeps them feeling as if, in spite of their toughness, they were still feminine and appealing.

I don't know about "feminine" and "appealing," I told Fiona, but

I do know this: Money has always made me nervous. I could never let too much of it build up. Whenever cash began to accumulate in my checking account, I had a hard time letting it just sit there, seeming to demand something of me. A thousand, two thousand, and as if on cue, I would find a way to get rid of it. I tried to spend wisely, buying good prints and books and theater tickets, investing in a cultured life, but considering the effect on my security, I might as well have been blowing it all at The Limited.

WHEN I split up with my children's father years ago, he was ill and unable to help with their support; thus, as a young single mother, I never had quite enough to meet the bills. As a midlife mother of teenagers who was finally earning a decent living, I tried to make it up to them—private schools, Tony Lama boots, the latest Rollerblades. I spent more on them than I should have, more than I could afford, really, since I wasn't investing consistently in my Keogh account. Buying nice things for my kids gave me momentary zaps of power, but I can see now that spending without any plan was undermining the deep feeling of pride and maturity I would have developed had I really been taking care of myself.

I had a bookkeeper to pay my bills and keep track of my expenses. I rationalized that this saved my precious time for earning a living, but as I became more removed from the details of my financial situation, I became distanced from its reality. My bookkeeper would tote up how much I'd spent each month, and each month I'd be surprised. But immediately I'd think, "Thank God there's enough there to cover all the bills." Never mind that the bills were far too high. Spending, I'd tell myself, was what expansive, self-respecting people did. I knew how to take care of myself. I knew how to take care of my property. How free it felt not to have to compromise on household repairs, landscaping, and improvements. I ordered bluestone retaining walls built (presumably to protect against erosion). I had my outside studio Sheetrocked. Then I decided I didn't like trudging across the snow to my studio in the winter and built a huge office in the house, combining two bedrooms and knocking through the attic to create a soaring ceiling. It's where I work, after all, I said.

The room was great for working, the best I'd ever had, although I'm sure I could have accomplished the same effect on much less if I'd planned. I never planned. To plan felt constricting, as if I were putting limits on myself. I hated limits. I felt I'd been living all my life with constraints. In my late forties I wanted to feel strong and invincible, so I barely noticed that my income wasn't quite what it had been. And after my relationship broke up, my expenses in that big house doubled. I knew intellectually what was happening, but I didn't allow myself to **really** *get* it. And so I made no change in my spending habits. I just kept . . . spending.

Until one month there wasn't enough, and I made my first premature withdrawal from my Keogh in order to pay my bills. A little here, a little there, and before long I was owing heavy penalties and interest to the government. Here was the truth: I didn't want to have to manage my money. I would work like a dog if need be, and I did— anything to avoid making a plan and a budget and monitoring myself like someone who has a future to contend with.

My burgeoning financial crisis was one of the most difficult struggles of my midlife transition. As I worked toward resolving it, I began to feel better grounded, more in control, more confident about the future. Earning money is not enough, I finally understood. You have to rein it in and make it work for you.

Before you hit fifty, it's difficult to imagine a time when you'll no longer be in your prime, when you'll have bouts of illness, down times—periods, God forbid, when you may not be working. But at fifty, we are forced to look differently at the future. We see people becoming ill and dying. We see people losing jobs. Professionals who've had careers for years find themselves out on the street and don't get rehired. We see older women being "eased out" of their positions because they're thought no longer to *look* the part.

And we take stock.

A kind of I've-paid-my-dues mentality can hit us at this time of life. We want to take our vacations and buy our clothes. We want the best for our children and are thrilled to be in a position to offer them help. But to lay out a plan and accept limits now, so that we can be protected in the future—that's something else.

Getting serious about earning, investing, and planning for retirement can make us anxious, as if it were forcing us to acknowledge certain unpleasant truths about our current state of affairs. But if we face—and move past—the anxiety, we can gain new flexibility in our lives. With money of our own and a solid investment plan, we can become free to pursue the dreams we shelved earlier to raise our children. And we can liberate ourselves from our fear of being poor, isolated, and dependent in old age—a fear that diminishes the quality of our lives right now.

CHAPTER IX

NEW CHOICES

MOVING OFF FROM THE FRONTIERS OF FIFTY

Feeling Stuck • One Month in Boulder •
A Woman Reinvents Her Life • Still Creative After All These Years •
Unblocking • Jumping Off • "This Is Day One" • New Choices •
Who I Am Now Is the Matriarch

"I KEEP READING about these fifties women who are making big leaps and major changes, but it's hard for me to imagine a new hair color at this point. Everything seems preordained."

This is Fiona speaking. The Mamas call her their truthsayer because she often says the things we feel before we have the nerve to face them. "I had my shot at marriage and family and being needed all the time by everyone, and now it seems like I'm consigned to live out my days alone. When I looked at my garden this evening, I actually had the thought, 'But who's it for?' The only person who's seen it besides me this summer is Helen. Once. This strikes me as pathetic."

Fiona is beginning to panic. Trapped in the eye of her midlife transition, she feels no thrilling tumult, only the stranglehold of inertia.

FEELING STUCK

THE shift from early adulthood to midlife is major, according to Bertram Cohler; it is one of three "transformative periods" that require tremendous effort. Earlier shifts are the transformation from early to middle childhood (the five-to-seven shift) and the adolescent shift, which usually lasts into early adulthood. During such periods, says Cohler, we are particularly susceptible to feeling fragmented. It's as if we aren't really free to swing, to enter the new, until we let go of what was. In the meantime, we're not sure what works anymore.

The way we maintain coherence during times of change is by reformulating our life stories to accommodate a newly integrated sense of ourselves. It is for the most part an unconscious process. Fiona, without being aware of it, is in the midst of such a transformation. In restructuring her story, she will forge new connections between her life as it is now, her life when she was younger, and her future.

But in the meantime, though she has friends, financial security, and a career in real estate that's always treated her well enough, she feels agitated, as if something's awry. Her children are grown and gone, and becoming a "nonmother," as she puts it, has created for her a momentous change. She misses the gratification she got from being a mother. It's not that she *wants* to go on mothering for the rest of her life, for God's sake, but rather that a sense of the shape of her life that she always took for granted is now under siege. She's finding it hard to take up the clay of her daily existence and give it new form. "The summer's almost over, and I haven't *had* a summer," she complains. "Two bike rides, one walk up the mountain, no swimming, no dancing, no concerts."

So get off your butt and do something, the Mamas have begun saying. *Jump in. Mix it up.*

To Fiona, it doesn't feel quite that simple. Her mind is cluttered with the same obsessive litany: *Should I try something new, or is it too late? Should I move someplace else, or would I be miserable without my friends?* But the lack of change, the feeling of being understimulated, is getting to her. "It's a ridiculous way to live," she announces one day, stabbing out one of the cigarettes she must give up (along with every-thing else, she thinks ruefully).

Fiona is beginning to face the fact that she has to make a new life, but the familiar residue of dependency remains, with its telltale resentment. *After all I've done in my life, I have to change, and risk, and grow once again?*

Yes, once again. At least once again.

"As I was waking from my role-wrapped sleeping self, I realized I *knew* who I had been as a mother, as a wife, and as a daughter and as a sister," said Marilyn Mason, reviewing her experience for therapists at a Miami conference of the American Association for Marriage and Family Therapy. "But who was I now? Who was I inside?"

Part of our unsettled feeling comes from questioning whether what we're doing has value. This often becomes a concern of women who've spent most of their adult lives parenting. With the mother role gone, we feel the need to be doing something equally important, equally committed. But it won't descend upon us the way a child does, suddenly *there,* demanding everything we've got. It needs to be sought out, figured out, gone after.

For a while, like Fiona, Marilyn Mason felt miserably stuck. What she came to understand, she told the therapists attending the Miami conference, is that to get unstuck, she had first to come "unglued." That doesn't mean going crazy—it means enduring a limbo period of uncertainty. It means floundering, questioning, stay-ing up late staring at the moon, and wondering why everything feels so damnably unsettled, and what, if any, possible good can come of it.

It may also mean simply striking out for a new experience, any-thing that might jolt us out of the rut that can come of too many should-I's.

One Month in Boulder

Martha, a psychotherapist who has lived in Atlanta most of her life, went through a struggle much like Fiona's. I met her at a point when she was coming to some resolution of her internal crisis.

Long married to a man who'd become increasingly preoccupied with business, Martha found herself feeling stifled and constrained. She decided to spend a month at Naropa, a Buddhist institute in Boulder, Colorado, taking painting classes and meditating. It was her forty-ninth summer. She rented a cottage for a month and soon found her temporary respite in Boulder to be freeing. Not only freeing but *social*. "By the last week, I was being invited to parties and dinners. My husband said on the telephone, 'You haven't been home one night this week.' He wasn't jealous, just . . . surprised."

Before Boulder, Martha had had a dream in which she shared a new office with her friend Beverly, another therapist. In this dream office "there was art everywhere, magnificent, huge canvases," she told me. "The primary color was that Mediterranean blue, very powerful. And there were young people hammering up things. We had a clinical psychologist visiting us, and when I saw her coming up our walk, I thought, 'Oh god, what is she going to think of this?' She was an academic person, you know."

The "academic person" represented the strict, self-censoring side of herself, Martha thought, the side that had always been made anxious by the creative and free. But she *wanted* the creative and free.

The fall following her month in Boulder Martha attended a conference in Houston with Beverly. One morning, as they were in the hotel room getting dressed, her friend said, "I keep thinking of that dream you had, Martha. I wish we could practice together."

And suddenly Martha thought, *"Yes!"* For eight years she'd been in an office with five men (clinical psychologists, it's interesting to note). The time had come to move.

She and Beverly decided to buy a building that would house their offices and provide extra space in which they could expand their lives. "It's an old house, and we fixed it up. It's very homey, very nonsterile, very nonoffice. I paint there now. I have a watercolor studio. And Beverly's beginning to write. She's just created a writing room for herself. And of course we have our two offices. It's really emerging into this space where all kinds of unexpected things are happening."

Martha is still examining her midlife process, but she feels that what's going on with her is organic and positive. She writes in her journal. She paints. She practices her therapy. She watches her evolving relationship with a husband she has loved for many years and sees that as she is changing, so is he. There is about this woman a sense of coming into her own. She's not rebelling against anything—she's expanding, *getting,* soaking life up like a sponge.

Asked what she thinks about most often at this juncture, Martha grows animated. "Something is changing. I said to Beverly, in the spring, 'I really feel I'm being called up to *do* something, to make a change. I don't know what it is, but I'm excited about it.' And that's different for me. Instead of being fearful—'Oh my god, I'll have to make another change' or 'Something's going to be required of me, can I do it?'—the feeling is, 'I wonder what it's going to be? And where will it take me? And who will I meet along the way?' "

A WOMAN REINVENTS HER LIFE

SOMETIMES it's a dream we have, a film we see, a story we read that triggers the sense that anything is possible. When I was feeling my most stuck, wondering if and how I would ever make of my life something new, I came across the story of a woman who pushed out into a whole new realm after being stricken, young, with the death of her husband.

When she was fifty, Evelyn Nef thought her life was over. "I was recently widowed; my job had been phased out because of my husband's death, and I was moving to a new city to start all over again," she told sociologist Lydia Bronte. "Little did I know that the best years of my life were still ahead of me."

Nef was 49 the year her husband died. Her work, all those years, had been helping him with his academic research. After he died, Nef was surprised to be offered a job as executive assistant of the American Sociological Association, even though she was not a sociologist. A colleague at Dartmouth, believing in her administrative abilities, had made the offer.

Nef thought she might as well accept the job, which would require a move to Washington, though she felt as if she were "marking time." It would turn out that she had barely begun to tap into her emotional and intellectual resources.

Shortly after arriving at her new job in Washington, Nef met and fell in love with a history professor. This man was older, and since she was likely to outlive him, she knew she needed a profession. Though by now she was in her early sixties, she wanted to become a psychotherapist. The possibility that training institutes wouldn't be thrilled about accepting her was worrisome, but she lined up an interview with the director of the Institute for the Study of Psychotherapy, in New York.

Nef was admitted to the program. Ordinarily the Institute required a master's degree in social work. She didn't have one, but her research background, it turned out, counted for something. For three years, she commuted to New York, and after she graduated, she set up a practice in Washington. From the outset, she found the work exhilarating. "I think it was an advantage for me to start very late, because I have the feeling I don't have seven years on the couch to give to somebody. If I'm going to do this, I have to do this quickly. My patients solve their problems and move on."

In her late seventies and still at it, at the time when Bronte interviewed her for the Long Careers Study, Nef reported being energized by her work. When people asked her if seeing six or eight patients in a day wasn't exhausting, she said no. "I'm exhilarated because I've resolved, because I've helped, because the feedback is very good when you are successful as a therapist."

After forty years of exploring a range of interests and abilities, this woman had sprung herself into a career that perfectly suited her. Reading about Evelyn Nef gave me pause. Here, very definitely, was another Choice Point. I had been interested in psychotherapy since I was twenty years old and read Theodore Reich's *Listening with the Third Ear*. I had spent years in my own therapy, first in groups and then in analysis. I had written about psychological issues for years. Something had begun percolating in me, though I wasn't sure what.

We can become enervated when we're in a quagmire of "stuckness." I had worried that my draggy feeling might be due to age. Forget that I had had these periods of feeling stuck, and their concomitant lethargy, when I was younger. Doubts were popping up to undermine my confidence, left over from an earlier concept of "middle age" that I'd unwittingly been applying to my own life. *You fool,* I'd think, *look at your mother, winding down her life at 87. That's only thirty years away! Better get prepared for it now. Better think about cutting down, not looking to take on more. Get real. Give it up. Settle.*

I knew, at the same time, that my doubts were defensive, the very arguments against life that intrude whenever we're facing change. Still, I had concerns: Would my *juice* for moving into a new endeavor, my creativity, continue to stand me in good stead? Or would I dilute the creative energy I needed for writing by spreading myself too thin?

STILL CREATIVE AFTER ALL THESE YEARS

PSYCHOLOGIST Dean Keith Simonton of the University of California, who has studied creative people over time, says that although creativity may begin to decline gradually at this time of life, the decline is mild. Even when it reaches its lowest point, late in life, our creativity will still be *far higher* than it was earlier in life. What falls off, Simonton says, is quantity—the number of products, that is, not their quality. Thus, the woman who, like Evelyn Nef, decides to become a therapist in her sixties may find, in her eighties, that she has to cut down the size of her practice, but her interventions will likely be as brilliant as ever, if not more so.

In her Long Careers Study, Lydia Bronte found that almost half her subjects had shown a major peak of creativity beginning at about the age of fifty that in many cases lasted another twenty-five or thirty years. What emerged from their life stories was "an affirmation of the increasing richness of experience over time, of a deeper sense of identity, of a greater self-confidence and creative potential that can grow rather than diminish with maturity."

It was reassuring to me to learn, when I interviewed Gretchen Cryer about life in her fifties, that the energy she devoted to starting a brand-new business hadn't cut off her creative juices. If anything, the charge she got from her entrepreneurial venture fed her creativity.

After four years, Gretchen hired a professional manager to keep The Extended Family operating, then reinvolved herself in playwriting. When I spoke with her, she had just gotten a producer for an ambitious new musical. Based on the life of Eleanor Roosevelt, the play's story line is rooted in the intellectual maturity that Gretchen had developed during the twenty years since *I'm Getting My Act Together and Taking It on the Road.* For the new show, she read biographies and assimilated the history of the Roosevelt era to produce something dramatic, insightful, and fresh.

Gretchen and her partner Nancy Ford (their collaborations date back to college) were inspired by Rhoda Lerman's *Eleanor,* a fictionalized account of the year Eleanor discovered that her husband was having an affair with Lucy Mercer. "We came up with the idea of having it be about a birthday party Franklin throws for Eleanor, a hundredth birthday party, after they're all dead. It's being thrown by Franklin because Franklin hasn't seen her since the day he died with Lucy Mercer in his arms. He wants to make amends, so he's throwing Eleanor a big birthday bash at The Cosmos Club, and he's asked Alice to be the hostess. Alice, who never liked Eleanor, has invited the *world* to this party."

The "world" is the people who come to the theater to see the play. Alice has also invited all the controversial characters from Eleanor's past—including Lucy Mercer and Earl Miller (Eleanor's chauffeur in the years when Franklin was governor of New York, long after his affair with Lucy began and with whom she probably had an affair). Alice also invited Lorena Hickok, the Associated Press journalist who was desperately in love with Eleanor.

Gretchen is animated as she talks about this elegant woman whose intellect and creativity are bursting forth at midlife, after being restrained by her role as the good wife earlier in life. "In the 1920s, Eleanor got involved with this whole group of women, lesbians, union activists, they were all talking about women's rights. It opened Eleanor's eyes, and she became an activist."

Until he died, Eleanor never knew that Franklin had continued his affair with Lucy. "She'd made a deal that she would stay with him if he promised never to see Lucy again." When she first learned of the affair, "she'd wanted to leave him, but 'Mama' said if she left him, it would ruin his career." Eleanor didn't want that on her conscience. Instead, they set up an arrangement, Gretchen continued, by whose terms she owed him nothing from the point when she found out about Lucy.

Eleanor would never have gained her intellectual and political independence, Gretchen believes, had she remained the deferential wife. "Ultimately, that is the point of our theater piece. If Franklin hadn't betrayed Eleanor by falling in love with someone else—and he was really in love, Lucy Mercer was no bimbo, she was a very intelligent, lovely woman—if Franklin hadn't done that, Eleanor probably would have remained the deferential wife forever. She would *never* have gone out to trade and women's meetings in the 1920s. She never would have been radicalized."

"Sounds like Gretchen Cryer," I said, recalling the marriage breakup that had released her own creativity.

"Yes," she said, smiling. "I hadn't thought of that."

UNBLOCKING

THROUGHOUT the life course, we have developmental "reserves" that we draw on in times of challenge, when we must make major changes. No matter what our age, if we use these reserves to meet new challenges, we can expand our range of functioning. But at times, the process of change can be agonizingly slow and anxiety-producing. Is there something we can do to move it along more quickly?

Finding other women who've already undergone major life changes can be inspiring. In the course of discussing another matter entirely, I found out that a woman I had just met, small, feisty Bernice Cassady, had successfully negotiated a major change at midlife.

"There's something universal about becoming older, and *facing* having the option to choose," she told me. "That option to choose seems to also bring with it a responsibility, because of the feeling that we're not going to have many more times to choose. You go through all this yammer, yammer, yammer in your head. 'I don't want to waste this precious time. Now. It's now. If I louse up this precious opportunity that I didn't even know I'd *have* . . .' Well, after going through an awful lot of back and forth and soul-searching, I really came to grips with something. If I just take my self and *go* with it and *trust* myself, if I can just get to that place, then I'm smart enough to know that if I enter a field that's interesting to me, that I'm drawn to, I can make out of that something that will work for me."

Bernice had spent thirty years in personnel, becoming general manager of the recruitment firm she worked for and eventually starting her own firm. But she'd been interested in aesthetics all her life and had never gotten the chance to develop it. At sixty, she began taking courses at the New York School of Interior Design. "My first course was Historical Styles. I loved it. It didn't say to me, 'You're going to be a designer,' but it started teaching me things. Then I took a course in materials. I learned drafting and how to do blueprints. This year I'm taking a course in Visual Principles. It's about *seeing* things differently, about how to structure space differently."

And she just began work with her first client, a woman who wants her house redesigned. She's left her old business and is undertaking the construction of a design studio in her house in the country.

How did Bernice get past the "yammer, yammer, yammer" and move on? I wanted to know, since such incessant self-questioning seemed to be my own biggest hurdle.

"Don't try to decide what you're going to *be*. It's not about 'What am I going to *be*?' Or 'What am I going to do with *my life*?' That's the trap that you're dealing with," she told me (and she didn't even *know* me). "Your shoulds. Your perfection goals. Your doubts. Fears. Concerns. Your private voices. This is not about what you're going to *be*, it's about going through a process. It's okay not to have all the answers. To have the questions is important."

The first thing you must do, says psychologist Lawrence LeShan, is to make a commitment to yourself to find out what you want to do. One has to make room for the process of self-discovery. LeShan suggests beginning by doing something you want to do—it can be anything—at least once a week. Set aside a specific time for it. Maybe during that put-aside time, you'll take a walk, or have a massage, or go to a concert. But whatever it is, you have to *commit* the time. It may soon turn out you're not so interested in walking anymore. That's fine, says LeShan. The point is to tune in to yourself. The process may seem laborious in the beginning, but the very act of working at finding out what *you* like to do will make your inner voice begin striking a firmer note.

JUMPING OFF

THE first time I talked to her, in the spring of 1992, Carol was on the verge of pulling up stakes in Wisconsin. "I've got an M.F.A., a Ph.D., and I've been a university teacher in theater and drama since 1965. But I've burned out on academe. It doesn't challenge me. So I decided to get out and change my life."

A lesbian who was not in a relationship and has no children, Carol had won a battle with breast cancer and was now nine years cancer-free. She felt empowered by her hard-won health. But at 54, she felt that age was a definite issue. If she were going to pursue a new career, it would have to be now. "I want to move to L.A. and find my way into professional theater. I want to work on a different level. I want to develop my playwriting and just sort of push out in a new direction in the field that I've been with all these years."

In April, a month after I talked to her, Carol took a sabbatical and left Wisconsin for Los Angeles. Her first question was how she would support herself while she was starting something new. She had $130,000 in a retirement fund that had to stay put until she was 62.

She'd sold her house and put the money she'd made into a savings account, which she hoped she wouldn't have to touch. She needed to learn how to do something practical, some no-brainer skill she could use for immediate money. "When I stopped teaching, I said, 'Wait a minute. I don't have any skills. This is ridiculous—I can't *do* anything!' So I went to H&R Block's income tax school and took this intense course from hell in tax preparation."

She thought she would use the season with H&R Block as an internship, then go into business for herself. But the money that year was rock bottom—minimum wage plus 20 percent of her fees. "If you're not fast, it doesn't amount to much."

Still, she figured that getting by financially and being able to work in the theater at night were all she needed. She didn't care whether people thought her successful or unsuccessful. "I don't need approval the way I used to. I'm more able to do what I want to do and express what I want to express and behave the way I want to behave."

On the other hand, Carol feels she's a late bloomer. "If I'd had role models growing up, I think I would have done much better in terms of finding myself earlier and feeling that it's all right to be the way you are and not feel weird, and odd, and different."

In the 1960s, when Carol was beginning her career, there were no women playwrights or directors. "The only women in the theater were actresses, and that wasn't really what I wanted to do, which is why I ended up being a college professor."

But by the 1990s things had opened up for women in the theater business, and Carol wanted her chance. She was willing to give up her $50,000 a year teaching salary and hole up in a hot, windowless office plugging away at people's income tax forms because at night she had a stage and a darkened theater, and she was directing the actors from a seat in the audience. It wasn't long before she joined a directors' festival where most of her colleagues were in their twenties and thirties and just starting out.

Although she found her new life exciting and was proud of herself for taking the plunge, the reality of her move began hitting home within months. Working day and night, poor, and having to build a social network from scratch—it began to feel like more than she could cope with.

Close to two years after she arrived in L.A., I spoke to her again. "The bottom line," she told me two minutes into the conversation, "is that I'm not earning a living."

"You mean in the theater?"

"Right. The way these directing fees go, I'd probably have to do twenty shows a year to support myself. You catch me at a time when I have a major decision to make because the university wants me to come back. Last fall I said, 'No, no, I never want to come back.' But this year it all feels much harder, and if I don't make the decision to return, they're going to hire somebody else."

Carol was up against it. She'd have liked more time, but there *wasn't* more time. She was being forced to face the limitation imposed upon her by age. "If I were thirty years old, there wouldn't *be* any decision. But to pull this off you've got to have the kind of energy to be able to do a full-time job and do the theater work too. That's what it takes. One of the best directors in L.A. is a cab driver."

It wasn't that she hadn't put out energy. "I hit the ground running when I got here, and I've been going ever since. But now I'm figuring, 'How long can I keep doing this?' There are times when I say to myself, 'Shit, why aren't I thirty years old?' I could knock this place around. Give me five years, and I'll knock it around. But give me five years *now,* and I'll be sixty."

A week later Carol made her decision: She was going to return to her teaching post. "I've been plugging away for a year and a half, and it's been like starting over again. Starting from the bottom would be okay if I were thirty-five, but at this point I realize it would take more time and sacrifice than I'm willing to give."

Nevertheless, she feels positive about her experiment. "I don't see the decision to return to teaching as the easy way out. I gave it a try here, and if something had happened fast, that would be one thing. But nothing's happening fast, and it's clear to me, it takes time for anybody."

All of this—beginning with her decision to sell her house to get money to back up a new profession in a new place—was far from the easy way out. It revealed reserves of energy and creativity she may never otherwise have experienced. Deciding finally that she needed to preserve her energy and financial reserves and go back to the university was not a defeat, any more than Ulysses returned in defeat. It had been an adventure. The woman who met the world in her H&R Block tax office and directed theater productions was not the same teacher who'd left the university two years before. Nor would she ever conduct her life in quite the same way. She had touched depths in herself that safety circumscribes.

There were those, back in Wisconsin, who no doubt thought Carol's move to L.A. was crazy. "What was she trying to prove?" they asked. Stigmas are especially pernicious against aging women. We are supposed to stay narrow, safe, and conventional—and let the men have the adventures.

CAROLYN Heilbrun believes that the courage that manifests at fifty is a "uniquely female" phenomenon, a part of the power of our prime. It can be seen not only in those who, like Martha, break out of a dutiful wife role to become women on their own at fifty, but in mold-breakers like neurosurgeon Frances Conley, M.D., who earlier in her career may have had to behave like "one of the boys" but at fifty was no longer up for the game.

At midlife, something hit home. In 1991, tired of twenty years of harassment from her male colleagues, of being called "hon" in the operating room and having her legs fondled under the table during surgery, Conley quit her job as a neurosurgeon at the Stanford University Medical Center. Since she had never liked the comments about her body, for years she had dressed to hide it. "When you dress attractively and someone says something about the size of your chest, what are you going to say back—'I notice you've got a pretty good lump in your pants'?"

When Conley quit, she didn't crawl off like a victim but made plain and public the reasons for her decision. In so doing, she triggered a huge debate about harassment at the medical center and other academic institutions. Women in medicine came forth in droves to complain of harassment by male doctors and researchers. Conley spoke to the press, alerting the entire country about what had happened and why she'd made her decision.

Then Stanford, chastened, admitted its male doctors needed "education" about their behavior and invited her back with promises of a change. Frances Conley returned, holding her head high.

"This Is Day One"

Women find that midlife is a time when latent talents can be put to use in new directions. Such "adaptive competence," some researchers believe, is a mark of successful aging.

Margaret's siege with hysterectomy, for example, empowered her. She began looking for a job with more responsibility and, she was able to admit, more power. It wasn't just the brand-new bachelor's degree. Margaret knew that she could promote her life experience, and the knowledge transformed her. This time she was going for executive director of development for a large hospital.

"I went into these interviews, and I just did and said the most amazing things. I did not give a damn if they offered me this job. Before, I'd always felt like, 'Oh, I would be so lucky if I got this.' This time around I felt like they would be lucky to get me."

In her final interview with the board of directors, Margaret had—and acted on—a brilliant insight about power. "I looked around the table and I thought, 'This is a whole new ball game, kiddo. This is the beginning. This is Day One. This is Moment One. You can be in control of this thing. You have the power, you're a forceful person. You can take control of this interview right now, and they'll never get it back from you. Or you can let *them* have the power, and you'll never get it.' "

The woman who was head of the board liked her—Margaret knew that much. They'd had a four-hour lunch together. But now here were all these older guys, men from an earlier generation. "One of them looked down his long nose at me and said, 'You know, our previous executive director was a member of the Lions Club. We think it's important for the executive director to be in the community and to be part of these service clubs. Would you consider joining the Lions Club?'

"I said, 'Absolutely not. I wouldn't be caught dead in the Lions

Club. I'm very sorry. I'm sure they're friendly, nice people, but no, I wouldn't do that.' Well, their mouths just dropped. They weren't horrified, they were stunned."

Approaching fifty—and "one uterus later," as she puts it—Margaret could no longer play the go-along girl. "Someone piped up and said, 'That's an interesting answer. I always thought it was stupid that Barry was racing around to all these meetings and giving away his good information. I kind of wondered why he spent so much time doing that.' "

They liked her, that much soon became clear. The time had come to discuss money. "You get to a certain stage in life, and you have a number in mind," Margaret said to me. "Well, what they offered me was *not* the number. I said, 'No, it's not enough. I'm worth this other number. This is the number I want, and I don't care how you give it to me. Give it to me in dollars, give it to me in benefits, however you want to work it out. But that's the number.' The head of the board said, 'I'll call you back.' "

They threw a car lease into the pot, thereby producing the number Margaret wanted. But that wasn't the end of it. After hiring her, they told her they wanted her to lease a Ford. " 'It's an image thing,' they told me. 'We have to be careful what kind of image you have in the community, and that's why we always have our directors drive Fords.' I said, 'Look, that's not my image.' I said, 'You had no idea when you hired me what kind of car I drive. I could drive a red Maserati. I could drive a pickup.' I said, 'Do you mean to tell me that once you've hired me, you feel you can tell me what kind of car to drive?' "

The car she had been planning to buy the next time around was a Miata, and that was the car she wanted now. "I'll compromise," Margaret told them. "I won't get the red, I'll get the white."

In the past, during such negotiations, Margaret would soft-pedal what she wanted. "I never wanted to ask for too much. Holding out for that last few thousand dollars with the hospital board made me very nervous. It was like saying, 'I deserve this. You must give it to me.' "

"You were going the whole way with it," I said.

"No compromise. I want what I want."

"And 'I'm *worth* what I want.' "

"And I'm worth what I want. And they gave it to me! I beat out sixty-five other people for this job. I feel pretty good."

She is also driving a white Miata.

Power no longer felt "unwomanly." Driving a sports car and asserting her needs and self-worth felt womanly. "Womanly as hell," says Margaret.

NEW CHOICES

WILLA and I have retreated to a spot in the mountains with a 360-degree view. You have to cross a little stream in the woods to get there. Often empty, Magic Meadow, as it's known, is a place under a huge sky to talk and to wonder, to try and come to grips. Women our age need such places. Women our age need one another.

"Fifty-five feels much older than turning fifty felt," says Willa, prying open the basket with our lunch. "It's halfway through the decade, and this is supposed to be the Big Transitional Decade. I feel like I haven't made the transition."

I nod. "This has been a kind of a crisis year for me," I say, "with my father dying, and me going back into therapy. I think I need to make a new life for myself. A patch here and a patch there isn't going to do it. It feels like I need a major change."

"You've been talking about moving back to the city for I don't know how long," says Willa. "Almost since you and R. split up."

It's true. I lived in New York for years in my twenties and thirties and loved it, but who knew if I'd like it now? I've been temporizing. "I think I'm afraid of losing something if I move back. I'm afraid of being in this new place, and not knowing anybody, and not being able to make a life."

I'm discovering that it's going to take an effort on my part, and courage. Life isn't just going to slide slowly and gracefully into something new and wonderful.

Deer come to the edge of the woods, look at us, and turn back. We are sitting near an old campfire and the air smells of woodsmoke.

Willa breaks off a hunk of baguette. "I think I've been taking the path of least resistance, focusing everything on my work and not really admitting that I feel lonely and understimulated. I've had these ideas, you know, about going back to school."

"For?"

"For nothing. For me. I mean, I wouldn't even *care,* I would want to do it just to learn, to study in some sort of systematic way."

It seems like a productive idea, a perfectly sane idea, but Willa has been harboring this notion for several years, turning it over and over in her mind, but never sending off for a catalog, much less trying a course. "Why is it so easy just to sit, letting the good ideas drift by?" she asks.

"Maybe," I say, "you have to reach the point where you're really feeling uncomfortable, and are *aware* that you're feeling uncomfortable, and that it's *not fun,* before—"

"Before something changes."

"Before *you* change."

WILLA is quiet for a while, lying on her back and looking at the sky. "I think the whole thing has to get shaken up. I have to strike out for myself, consider all kinds of possibilities, really knock it open."

It occurs to me that since I got married and had kids, my whole life has been driven by outside forces.

"By the needs of others," says Willa.

It's true. Even though I began writing as a young mother, most of my life-shaping choices had to do with others—my man, my children, who they were, where they wanted to be, what kinds of lives they wanted to lead. Now, for the first time, the choices that will determine the shape and texture and tone of my life have only to do with me.

"When your life has always revolved around others, it takes a while to even begin to focus on yourself," Willa observes. "And once you start to get a glimpse of what it is you want, you have to actually create a new environment, a new set of priorities, to support it."

I've had a glimpse of what I'd like, but when it comes to making a new environment for myself, I have to acknowledge, I've been treading water. "For a long time I thought the Big Change was ending that sixteen-year relationship," I tell Willa. "That was it. That was the big gutsy thing to do when I was fifty."

"And it was."

"And it was. But it was only half the story."

"Right, and now you're dealing with the other half," she reminds me.

THE other half. That's the part that's new. There's a whole new stretch of adulthood to look forward to, and that's exciting.

At the same time, it's quite clear that it's the *last* stretch—which raises the stakes considerably.

"Once you become *conscious* of the fact that you're going to die eventually, it changes everything," says Willa.

When Willa was in her early forties she had difficulty with the idea of her own mortality. "It was as if I weren't going to die and I had all the time in the world. Now, ten years, twelve years later, it's different. I *feel* different. I feel serious about my life in a way I never did before. What I do now, the choices I make, have become much more important."

In the late 1980s, Carolyn Heilbrun wrote that women have retreated from the challenge and support of consciousness-raising that helped us define new lives for ourselves in the 1970s. We've gotten insular again, individualizing our experience to the point where we feel alone and inadequate. "Women," she wrote, "must turn to one another for stories. They must share the stories of their lives and their hopes and their unacceptable fantasies." It is through the telling and sharing of these things that we are able to transcend the more difficult parts of our histories and begin to reinvent our lives.

I pour some wine into the glasses we've stuck in the picnic basket. "There's a little cafeteria in this medical library I use," I tell Willa. "It's up on the fifth floor, this room with about six tables and a Puerto Rican guy who cooks food for whomever is in this really magnificent building, the New York Academy of Medicine. The place is always quiet. That day there were only two other people, two women, sitting at a little table in the back. I imagined they were doctors. While I ate my sandwich, I went on this fantasy about, What would it be like to be a doctor? What would it be like to be one of *them*? Those two women, I mean. The work I do can be isolating, you know. I'm always wondering what it would be like to—"

"To work with people."

"To be a psychoanalyst, actually. To work at an institute. Go to *meetings*."

We laugh. It occurs to me that this vulnerability I'm feeling, fantasizing about the conversation of those women and what their lives might be like in this big, secure, quiet academic building, is a function of my radar starting to get out there and shift around over dark waters. "The very fact that there are so many possibilities is unnerving," I say to Willa.

"But if you really gave yourself the luxury of getting into it," she replies, "who *knows* what you'd end up feeling about what you wanted to do or how you wanted to live."

People are constantly weaving together the threads of their lives in new ways so that they can give meaning to the past. But we're also trying to make sense of the events that are current in our lives, especially during times of change.

What had interested me at the New York Academy of Medicine Library was not the male doctors searching through medical journals; what had galvanized me was the two women in the cafeteria and wondering what their story might be. Carolyn Heilbrun says that as long as women are isolated from one another, not allowed to offer other women the most personal accounts of their lives, "they will not be part of any narrative of their own."

A narrative of my own. That is what it feels as if I'm trying to do right now, create my own story rather than have it be created for me by others. I am beginning to see that it involves a process, and that Willa and the rest of the Mamas are helping me with it.

It didn't take me long to recognize that I don't really want to become a psychoanalyst, or belong to an institute, or go to meetings; although allowing myself the fantasy worked me in the direction of finding out what I *do* want. What I need, what I long for, is less isolation, more affiliation. I want to keep writing, but from a broader base. I want to crack my life open.

Clouds scud by. The sun has started to lower itself into the tops of the pines. This conflict we are trying to talk our way through will not get resolved today; but we're beginning to get the picture, Willa and I, a sense of what it's going to take.

Who I Am Now Is the Matriarch

IN our fifties, there are possibilities that will not reveal themselves until we can accept and let go of the past, and take a chance on the future. Sifting through a huge box of family photographs recently, I was stunned into a kind of trance state from which I didn't emerge for several days. I felt myself to be the repository of all my family's memories. My mother had mailed me her albums—pictures of her parents, whom I had never met, pictures of herself and my father when they were young and in love, pictures of me when I was a month old. In the box, also, were my own family pictures, my children as infants, color "portraits" of them provided by the diaper company, my husband in his healthier years when he was flush with fatherhood, my husband in his later years, when the depression from which he suffered for so long, without knowing its name, suffused his face like a mask. Me in long hair and a miniskirt, dancing at a party with him. Me, a thin, thirteen-year-old girl in a skirted bathing suit, standing by the ocean with the wind blowing through my hair. My mother and my father in their later years—always, it seems, with an azalea bush in the background—their white hair, their advancing age. Actually, I recognize now, that age of theirs was advancing when they were *my* age.

It is all too much; these images and their memories weigh me down. It is as if I have never before had time to take them all in as a whole, to integrate them. This is my life!

And it is the life I have had whether I wanted it or not. I see, now, that along with all the other feelings, I also have the uncomfortable one of not having *chosen* this life, these people, the sepia-toned immigrant grandparents, my husband's parents, my mother-in-law's *father,* a man so removed from our lives and consciousness that only now, for the first time, do I see the unmistakable look of depression on his face. So it was not only on his father's side that my husband had this illness, I think; it was on his mother's, as well.

Depression, thinness, too little money: maybe, that day, it was simply a mood that made me see everything so negatively. Or perhaps I'd never seen it so of-a-piece before. Perhaps I'd never allowed myself that experience. The Pandora's box of those curling old snapshots, as in Sue Miller's *Family Pictures,* brought turmoil. Yes, there is dignity in the life of a family, but there is also tremendous struggle, and pain, and misunderstanding.

I know what this is, this weight—this burden, almost—of being the repository of all these memories! I have become the matriarch. It is to me that they look now, my children, my mother—even my father, still demanding that I give meaning to his life. These images fill my quiet house for two days like a malaise, a kind of doom. I cannot *believe* that I own all this, that I have all this to contend with, to face up to, to acknowledge: my brother's weddings, his wives that I never knew, my mother's brothers and sisters that I never knew, my own infancy and early childhood. It is all here in this box, and somehow I am responsible for it.

That's the odd part. When I look at the depressed face of my mother-in-law's father, whom I never met, I feel *responsible* for it. When I see my husband almost grimacing, toward the end, with the effort of containing an illness he didn't understand, I feel responsible. Now, years later, I know more about that illness than he ever did. *Knowing* makes me responsible.

No wonder I went all those years without quite looking at those pictures, not thinking about my mother's endless brothers and sisters, my brother's wives, my mother-in-law's father—not wanting to in some way have to deal with them. I had enough to deal with then. Now, in the relative calm of my fifties, I look, and I take them all in. They are mine, they are what I was dealt. These are my family, a substantial part of my world.

The one thing about which I feel no ambivalence is my children. Looking at the small, silly pictures of them when they were young, I remember the single-minded intensity with which I loved and cared for them. Sometimes I think I would like the chance to do it over again with them, to make it better, different, to be to them then who I am now.

Who I am now is the matriarch—strong, flexible, the repository of our family's dreams and failures, the knower of its secrets and illnesses, the one who survived it all, the Middle Woman who holds it all together. The sense of responsibility I feel is awesome. I am the glue, the earth, the mud of which it's made.

I don't believe this experience is unique. It has to do with both my age and my gender: I am a midlife woman, and I have a lot to account for, a lot to live up to, a lot of people to take care of, a lot, still, to *do* and be. Entering into that swirl of memory and pain was part of facing who I am. I think this is what shocked me most about going through the family pictures: It was an assault to the story I'd made up about who I was, the limits I'd placed on who would be allowed "inside" my world and who would have to stay out. All those curled and yellowing fragments (other women would have mounted and carefully framed their photographs, I was sure) now insist upon being allowed in. "We are part of it too," they say.

In letting them in, I have to change.

Important for psychological health is a sense that life has *continuity*. Yet that sense is actually something we make up. We structure and restructure our understanding of experience, processing new information in the light of what we've already learned. "The inner life of the mind," says Bernice Neugarten, "is like a river or a stream, one whose content gradually changes as it accumulates materials from the banks it has touched."

Sometimes I look in the mirror and see a girl. It's a trick of the evening, when the light slants through the window in a certain way, and for a moment, as I prepare to go out to the café for dinner, I am uplifted, steadied in the view of myself I have held for so long. But in the morning, with no makeup, my hair a mess, I rise up from having stooped to take in the cat and see myself tall in the hall mirror. There, before me, is the truth: I am a woman who has aged. I have to love myself this way if I am to love myself at all. I have to love the flabby stomach, the fine dry wrinkles, the skin that becomes itchy if I don't slap lotion on it several times a day. *This,* not the evening glamour, the new red lipstick, is me.

But isn't it funny. In allowing myself to really look at those old family photos, I was able to see some things for the first time. I saw that my father, in his youth, was a handsome man, and I had somehow never seen that before. Because I had always been told I looked like my father, seeing him in this way changed something. I saw that that girl on the beach, and the later one, at seventeen, was attractive. I had always thought otherwise. I had always believed that girl gaunt and gawky and even, in some sense, unworthy—that she didn't quite "pass." Now I am able to take her inside and cherish her.

It is because I forgave my father and allowed myself to love him before he died that I am able to see him differently now. My father is not who I thought he was, he is someone fragile and lovable, and in acknowledging that I have become able to love myself. That is something wonderful that has tumbled out of my midlife shake-up.

There would be others.

IN the summer of his eightieth year, my father and I were driving in the country after my daughter's college graduation. It was one of those spring days that obliterate the ravages of winter. My father said, sighing, " 'What is so rare as a day in June?' " I think of his ability to savor the moment as a saving bright spot in his complicated personality. He had a mind that was at home in quantum mechanics, ideas the rest of us could not grasp, much less talk with him about. Yet he had an eye for nature and the simple, good things of life. I think that that "eye" is one of the gifts of maturity. It doesn't come as a result of slowing down. It comes with acceptance.

But before that final acceptance, there must come, for women, acceptance of another kind. We must free ourselves of society's images of us to begin to accept ourselves.

With this will come new joy and energy and assertiveness. We can, like Frances Conley, assert ourselves, even if it means leaving a prestigious job at a prestigious institution.

We can, like Carol, sell a house and give up academe and take a job with H&R Block, just for the chance to direct shows off-off-Broadway.

We can, like Gretchen Cryer, take up a new career to increase our financial stability—and still pursue our creative lives.

As things fall into place (and I'm sure they'll fall out again, at some transition point in later years), I've come to accept my life, my past, the foolish moves I've made, the negative relationships I've entered—and stayed in, oh, how many years! I accept my bravado in the face of fear, my lack of courage in the face of risk. I accept what I have without looking for "closure," some magical endpoint at which everything is resolved, everything perfect. Nothing, in any ultimate sense, gets resolved; nothing closes. *Getting* this allows a new openness. And from this position, finally, I am able to move on.

A few months after my conversation with Willa in the meadow, I got an idea: I could lead groups for women who want to explore the psychological and social issues of midlife. I got excited about being involved with others who are in the same place in the life course, facing the same Choice Points. I thought I could take what I had been learning in my research and with the Mamas and bring it to others.

CAROLYN Heilbrun has noted that midlife is different for women than for men, who at this age may need to "discover new courage, perhaps, but need not profoundly change their lives, need not dedicate them to something new."

That dedication of our lives to something new is what links women together at fifty. It's what enlivens us and makes us different from the generations of women who came before. It is the point, and promise, of this new prime. Red Hot Mamas are on the cusp. We are changing the future for women once again.

EPILOGUE

GOING BACK

I AM MOVING back to the city, making my peace. I guess I'm never going to have an allée of tree hydrangeas; a hill swept with Siberian iris is beyond my capabilities. Something about living in the country never quite took hold, even though I stayed in it almost twenty years. I had pots of things on the patio—annuals, mostly, that I bought good and thriving each June. I had a country kitchen that, in these recent years, I hardly used, choosing to eat city style in my local café at night. In the summer I'd ride my bike, but guess what? I had to put it in the car and drive five or six miles to a safe place before I could ride it. The roads in my neighborhood were too mountainous, too unsafe.

In my head, always, I stayed a city girl. Anyone who knows me will tell you that. Still, it seems strange, retiring back to the city. Of course I am not retiring at all. I am starting off on the second half. I do not plan to remain in the holding pattern I've been in. Nor will I mourn the mountains and rutted country roads and hills of laurel. Returning to New York will fill me with a new fire.

But I have few illusions, having lived in the city for eighteen years, in the 1960s and early 1970s, a green girl right out of Catholic college who "roomed" with her old college friends, worked at a women's magazine, and finally married on the heels, as we did it in those days, of getting pregnant. I remember the rutty windowsills of the old floor-through in Chelsea, the crazed super who'd get drunk and sit in the basement in the corner where you took the garbage on weekend nights, threatening to set off a bomb at any moment. You just hoped he'd pass out. I remember the junkies on Eighth Avenue, the fights heard through thin walls, the screams and sighs of miserable people living too close.

We were writers, my husband and I. We lived like graduate students and raised our babies, all three of them born in that floor-through, with a breeze coming in through the fire-escape window in their bedroom. One night when we were away someone came in through that fire escape and robbed the apartment. Blackened newspaper torches lay on the hall floor. Drawers hung open, their contents flung quickly about. Nothing was missing, since we had nothing worth stealing, save a little gold medal blessed by the Pope that my first child's grandmother had given her.

Now, although my return to the city was haunted by old memories, I imagined it somewhat differently. After all, I have grown up in the intervening years, become a different person from when I first arrived, breathless, so glad to be away from the nuns, so entranced by the lack of rules or even guidelines. So terrified, really, of it all.

I want to go back to the Upper West Side, where I'd lived the last nine years of my Manhattan life, the children growing up in a playground in Riverside Park. That family neighborhood isn't such a good idea for now, but I like the idea of a park. Central Park is the obvious answer, Central Park, where I could take my bike and maybe even learn to Rollerblade. Oh, I have big notions.

Scanning the apartment ads week after week, I learn the lingo that describes what it is I am looking for: European-style one-bedroom with direct park views in a prewar building with doorman. I want the West Eighties, but I'll take the Nineties. I want high ceilings, dark floors, big old windows through which I can see clear to Fifth Avenue. (Will there be someone for me on the other side of the park, the way Woody was for Mia? Probably not. Probably I don't want anyone anyway. At least I don't want Woody.)

I want walls thick enough to shield me from the screams and sighs of others. I want a properly decorated tree in the lobby at Christmastime—none of those all-blue schemes for me. The way I figure it is this. I can use the big entrance gallery as my library, lining its walls with bookshelves. Either I'll use the bedroom as my office and sleep on a couch in the living room, or I'll keep the bedroom and set up my work space in the living room. Entertaining, after all, will be only occasional, and there are ways of getting around the problem. This space is to be for me, engineered for my life and no one else's.

And what of what I am giving up? They say you have to rehearse for change. My land upstate abuts a neighbor's land, forested and probably undevelopable. My own three acres lie on a kind of bluff above a trout stream. You can see small mountains and a steepled church from the back of my house, which used to be its front. The house is one of the few remaining Dutch frame buildings in the area, more than two hundred years old. There's a pond, of course, with birch trees hanging over it, and a small outbuilding down by the woods that I used to use as my studio when the kids were still around. The place is killer.

I've lived in it longer than I've lived anywhere else, going on eleven years. Some people would die for this, but my heart isn't in it. Walking by a bank on Park and Fifty-seventh around midnight, looking in at the people sleeping in the lit lobby, lying facedown, their foreheads resting on little pillows made of rolled clothing, Pepsi cans and lighters placed neatly by the sides of their heads, my heart is there.

Surely I sentimentalize, you say.

That may be, but I'm giving myself the chance to find out. In the meantime, here is where I'll continue to write, here is where I'll run my groups, here is where I'll pot my annuals, sticking them on a crumbly windowsill if need be. The point is, this is not the last chance. Nothing is written in stone. The point . . . is moving.

NOTES

CHAPTER I

page

13 "and willing to catch hell . . .": Lois W. Banner, in *In Full Flower: Aging Women, Power, and Sexuality* (New York: Alfred A. Knopf, 1992), cites Sara Evans, *Personal Politics: The Roots of Women's Liberation in the Civil Rights Movement and the New Left* (New York: Vintage, 1980), p. 51.

14 Orth quotes: Maureen Orth, "The Lady Has Legs," *Vanity Fair,* May 1993, p. 178.

15 Heilbrun quote: Carolyn G. Heilbrun, "How Girls Become Wimps," *The New York Times Book Review,* Oct. 4, 1992, p. 14.

CHAPTER II

21 Bronte quote: Lydia Bronte, *The Longevity Factor* (New York: HarperCollins, 1993), p. xv.

22 "you could reach fifty . . .": Ibid., p. xvii.

25 a trade-off for the loss of youthful vigor: Jon Hendricks and C. Davis Hendricks, *Aging in Mass Society: Myths and Realities,* 3rd ed. (Boston: Little, Brown & Co., 1986), p. 222.

25 Ryff quote: Carol D. Ryff, "Subjective Experiences of Life Span Transitions," *Gender and the Life Course,* ed. Alice S. Rossi (New York: Aldine, 1985), pp. 97–110.

25 Brim quote: Alice S. Rossi, "Aging and Parenthood in the Middle Years," in *Life-Span Development and Behavior,* ed. Paul B. Baltes and Orville G. Brim, Jr., vol. 3 (New York: Academic Press, 1980), p. 147.

25 "it seizes on astrology . . .": Ibid., p. 146.

26 "generativity," that presumed pinnacle . . . : Grace K. Baruch, Rosa-

lind C. Barnett, and Caryl Rivers, *Lifeprints: New Patterns of Love and Work for Today's Women* (New York: McGraw-Hill, 1983), pp. 1–10.

26 "The stage of life crucial for the emergence . . .": Alice S. Rossi, "Aging and Parenthood in the Middle Years," p. 184.

27 most people who've reached forty . . . : Bernice L. Neugarten, "The Awareness of Middle Age," in *Middle Age and Aging,* ed. Bernice L. Neugarten (Chicago: University of Chicago Press, 1968), p. 891.

28 Asked what age they'd pick . . . : Rossi, "Aging and Parenthood in the Middle Years," p. 184.

28 "often with a note of despair.": Ibid., p. 175.

30 Anderson quote: Anderson spoke at the conference "Treating Couples: Clinical Challenges in the 1990s," sponsored by Harvard Medical School, in Boston in October 1992.

31 "Women do not have the right . . .": William E. Schmidt, "Birth to 59-Year-Old Raises British Ethical Storm," *The New York Times,* Dec. 29, 1993, p. 1.

31 Carlson quote: Margaret Carlson, "Old Enough to Be Your Mother," *Time,* Jan. 10, 1994, p. 41.

31 Bateson quote: Bateson spoke at the conference "Conscious Aging," sponsored by The Omega Institute, in Manhattan in 1992.

32 Martin quotes: April Martin, "Dreams on Ice," *The New York Times Magazine,* Nov. 28, 1993, p. 46.

33 Rodin quotes: Maggie Mahar, "Making It in the Ultimate Men's Club," *Working Woman,* Mar. 1993, p. 64.

35 in adolescence something radical happened . . . : Carolyn G. Heilbrun, "How Girls Become Wimps," *The New York Times Book Review,* Oct. 4, 1992, p. 13. Heilbrun is reviewing *Meeting at the Crossroads: Women's Psychology and Girls' Development* by Carol Gilligan and Lyn Mikel Brown (Cambridge, MA: Harvard University Press, 1992).

35 Heilbrun quote: Ibid.

36 Foe quotes: Natalie Angier, "Drawing Big Lessons from Fly Embryology," *The New York Times,* Aug. 10, 1993, p. C1.

CHAPTER III

38 Barber quote: Clifton Barber, "Transition to the Empty Nest," *Aging and the Family,* ed. Stephen J. Bahr and Evan T. Peterson (Lexington, MA: Lexington Books, D.C. Heath and Company, 1989), pp. 1–32.

40 Parents in the "empty nest" phase . . . : F. H. Scherz, "Maturational Crises and Parent-Child Interaction," *Social Casework,* vol. 36 (1971), pp. 362–69.

42 Goldscheider quote: Jane Gross, "Divorced, Middle-Aged and Happy:

Women, Especially, Adjust to the 90s," *The New York Times,* Dec. 7, 1992, p. A14.

42 "Everything's always done . . .": Lawrence Kutner, "Parent and Child," *The New York Times,* Dec. 31, 1992.

43 Barbara Grizzuti Harrison, "Hers," *The New York Times,* p. 14.

44 gerontologist Elaine Brody found . . . : Elaine M. Brody, "Women in the Middle and Family Help to Older People," *The Gerontologist,* vol. 21, no. 5 (1981), pp. 471–80.

44 30 to 40 percent . . . : Ibid.

44 Sixty percent of adult daughters . . . : Abigail M. Lang and Elaine M. Brody, "Characteristics of Middle-Aged Daughters and Help to Their Elderly Mothers," *Journal of Marriage and the Family* (Feb. 1983), p. 196.

44 McGoldrick quote: Monica McGoldrick, "Women Through the Family Life Cycle," *Women in Families,* eds. Monica McGoldrick, Carol M. Anderson, and Froma Walsh (New York: W. W. Norton and Co., 1991), p. 202.

47 With over two-fifths of older people . . . : Brody, "Women in the Middle," p. 472.

48 By the time they reach 75 . . . : Lang and Brody, "Characteristics of Middle-Aged Daughters," p. 199.

48 twenty-three hours of parent care a week: Ibid.

55 In a 1991 study published by the Wellesley College Center for Research on Women . . . : Grace Baruch and Rosalind Barnett, "Adult Daughters' Relationships with Their Mothers," *Journal of Marriage and the Family,* vol. 45, no. 3 (Aug. 1993).

55 Barnett quote: Ibid.

55 *devote time equivalent to a full-time job.*: Lang and Brody, "Characteristics of Middle-Aged Daughters," p. 197.

55 "To an extent unprecedented in history . . .": Brody, "Women in the Middle," pp. 471–80.

56 McGoldrick quote: McGoldrick, "Women Through the Family Life Cycle," p. 204.

56 "They shop and run errands . . .": Ibid.

56 sons lack "responsibility or family feeling,": Ibid.

64 Woodman quotes: Woodman was speaking at the Omega Institute's conference, "Conscious Aging," held in Manhattan in 1992.

Chapter IV

71 Banner quote: Lois W. Banner, *In Full Flower: Aging Women, Power, and Sexuality* (New York: Alfred A. Knopf, 1992), p. 15.

74 Burstyn quote: In Cathleen Rountree, *On Women Turning Fifty* (Harper San Francisco, 1993), p. 16.

77 Yalom quote: In Susan L. Crowley, "The Sin of Aging," *AARP Bulletin,* vol. 32, no. 9 (Oct. 1991), p. 2.

78 Seligson quote: Marcia Seligson, "Can a Feminist Have a Facelift?" *Lear's* (Mar. 1992), p. 52.

82 Friedan quote: Betty Friedan, *The Fountain of Age* (New York: Simon and Schuster, 1993), p. 30.

82 In the few societies . . . : Pauline Bart, "Why Women's Status Changes in Middle Age: The Turns of the Social Ferris Wheel," *Sociological Symposium,* vol. 3 (Fall 1969), pp. 1–18.

83 Sontag quote: Maggie Scarf, "The Middle of the Journey," *Family Therapy Networker* (July/Aug. 1992).

84 "became shapeless figures . . .": Banner, *In Full Flower,* p. 296.

84 "In her drawings . . .": Ibid.

84 Wylie quote: Philip Wylie, *Generation of Vipers* (New York: Rinehart, 1942), pp. 186–87. Wylie's contribution to the negative view of aging women is described by Banner in ibid., p. 303.

84 Erikson quote: Ibid., p. 303.

85 "Ms. Kahn is 51.": Michael Specter, "Funny? Yes, But Someone's Got to Be," *The New York Times,* Apr. 8, 1993, p. C1.

85 Hopewell-Ash quote: Edwin Hopewell-Ash, *Melancholia in Every-Day Practice* (London: John Bale, 1934), pp. 41–42, quoted in Banner, *In Full Flower,* p. 295.

85 Zelda Popkin reported . . . : Ibid., p. 307.

86 "When a woman of 48 . . .": Dr. Walter Gallichan is the "conservative physician" Banner quotes on p. 293 of ibid.

86 de Beauvoir quote: Simone de Beauvoir, *The Second Sex* (New York: Vintage Books, 1989), p. 581.

88 Older women were sexually aggressive . . . : Havelock Ellis, *Studies in the Psychology of Sex,* vol. 1, *The Sexual Impulse in Women* (1905) (New York: Random House, 1942), p. 243, discussed in Banner, *In Full Flower,* p. 286.

88 These normal genital changes . . . : Ibid., p. 92.

88 "Nine out of ten erotomaniacs . . .": de Beauvoir, *Second Sex,* p. 581.

89 Gimmelson quotes: Deborah Gimmelson, "Pumped Up," "Hers" column, *The New York Times Magazine,* June 27, 1993, p. 16.

90 Scarf quotes: Scarf, "Middle of the Journey."

90 One 55-year-old lawyer: Ellen Cole, "Sex at Menopause: Each in Her Own Way," in *Women and Therapy,* ed. Ellen Cole and Esther Rothblum (Binghamton, NY: Haworth Press, 1988).

90 "One, if not *the* greatest blessing . . .": Barbara E. Sang, "Moving

Toward Balance and Integration," *Lesbians at Midlife: The Creative Transition* (San Francisco: Spinsters Book Co., 1991), p. 208.

91 a quarter of the women experienced . . . : Ibid., p. 209.

91 Posin quote: Robyn Posin, "Ripening," in *Lesbians at Midlife,* p. 144.

92 Hendricks quote: Jon Hendricks and C. Davis Hendricks, *Aging in Mass Society: Myths and Realities,* 3rd ed. (Boston: Little, Brown & Co., 1986), p. 275.

Chapter V

102 Carter quotes: Betty Carter, "Stonewalling Feminism," *Family Therapy Networker* (Jan./Feb. 1992), p. 64.

102 "stone wall against which we are stalled.": Ibid.

103 "accommodate the implacable . . .": Ibid.

107 Marital unhappiness peaks . . .: Martha Kirkpatrick, "Some Clinical Perceptions of Middle-Aged Divorcing Women," in *Divorce as a Developmental Process,* ed. Judith Gold (Washington, DC: American Psychiatric Press, 1988), p. 84.

107 Among those who are older . . . : Ibid., p. 83.

107 there were almost 1.5 million divorced . . . : Jane Gross, "Divorced, Middle-Aged and Happy: Women, Especially, Adjust to the 90s," *The New York Times,* Dec. 7, 1992, p. A14.

107 Between 1970 and 1988 . . . : Ibid.

108 "For the first time in my life . . .": Quoted in ibid.

108 Heilbrun quote: Carolyn G. Heilbrun, *Writing a Woman's Life* (New York: Ballantine Books, 1988), p. 88.

108 "viewed marriage as a vise . . .": Gross, "Divorced, Middle-Aged and Happy."

109 Goldscheider quote: Ibid.

109 Only 17 percent . . . : Judith Wallerstein, "Women After Divorce: Preliminary Report from a Ten-Year Follow-Up," *American Journal of Orthopsychiatry,* vol. 56, no. 1 (Jan. 1986), p. 68.

109 "It appears that divorce . . .": Ibid., p. 76.

109 "a striking rise in self-esteem . . .": Ibid.

109 divorced men often die . . . : Gross, "Divorced, Middle-Aged and Happy."

110 Wallerstein quote: Wallerstein, "Women After Divorce," p. 73.

110 "There are so many blobs in pants . . .": Quoted in Edith Nemy, " 'What? Me Marry?' Widows Say No," *The New York Times,* June 18, 1992, p. C1.

110 "I don't need a man . . .": Ibid.

111 Second marriages break up . . . : Betty Carter, "Remarried Families: Creating a New Paradigm," *The Invisible Well,* ed. Marianne Walters,

Betty Carter, Peggy Papp, and Olga Silverstein (New York: Guilford Press, 1988), p. 333.

112 Volk quote: Patricia Volk, "Strings Attached," "Hers," *The New York Times Magazine,* June 28, 1992.

112 Howard quotes: Margo Howard, "Jerks, Oddballs, and Egomaniacs," *Boston* magazine, May 1993.

113 Over 75 percent of men older than 65 . . . : Froma Walsh and Monica McGoldrick, "Loss and the Family Life Cycle," in *Family Transitions,* ed. Celia James Falicov (New York: Guilford Press, 1988), p. 327.

113 For every ten women between forty and fifty . . . : Ibid.

114 Goldscheider quote: Gross, "Divorced, Middle-Aged and Happy."

114 They got stuck in a transition . . . : Ibid.

114 In the fall of 1992 . . . end up losing themselves: Sonia Dimidjian's discussion of divorced women took place during a seminar called "After the Ball Is Over: Divorce and Midlife Women," at the American Association for Marriage and Family Therapy, in Miami in October 1992.

115 Ruch quote: Nemy, " 'What? Me Marry?' Widows Say No," p. C1.

115 Wilson quote: Gross, "Divorced, Middle-Aged and Happy."

115 Howard quote: Howard, "Jerks, Oddballs, and Egomaniacs," p. 66.

115 "the basic assumptions about the family as we know it": Sonia Dimidjian at the American Association for Marriage and Family Therapy conference, in Miami in October 1992.

116 Divorced women "are *not* willing . . .": Ibid.

116 "It allowed them . . . ": Ibid.

116 "I took my maiden name . . .": Ibid.

116 Lockwood quote: Gross, "Divorced, Middle-Aged and Happy."

116 Anderson quote: Anderson, "After the Ball Is Over: Divorce and Midlife Women."

117 Single women at midlife . . . : Sharon Hicks and Carol Anderson, "Women on Their Own," in *Women in Families,* ed. Monica McGoldrick, Carol M. Anderson, and Froma Walsh (New York: W. W. Norton & Co., 1991), p. 323.

119 Women are four times more likely . . . : Walsh and McGoldrick, "Loss and the Family Life Cycle," p. 327.

119 Each year, almost as many women . . . : Elaine M. Brody, "Women in the Middle and Family Help to Older People," *The Gerontologist,* vol. 21, no. 5 (1981), p. 477.

119 McGoldrick quote: Monica McGoldrick, "Women Through the Family Life Cycle," in *Women in Families,* eds. McGoldrick, Anderson, and Walsh, p. 214.

120 The story of Sara is told by Betty Carter in "Single Women: Later Years," in *Invisible Well,* eds. Walters, Carter, Papp, and Silverstein, p. 403.

121 Annette, Joan, Gina, and Marianne: Ibid.

121 Sara's quote: Ibid.

124 Carter quote: Betty Carter, "Divorce: His and Hers," *The Invisible Web,* ed. Marianne Walters, Betty Carter, Peggy Papp, and Olga Silverstein (New York: The Guilford Press), p. 256.

124 "to leave behind the ideas . . . .": Dimidjian, "After the Ball Is Over: Divorce and Midlife Women."

124 de Beauvoir quote: Simone de Beauvoir, *The Second Sex* (New York: Vintage Books, 1989), p. 471.

127 "Most single women . . .": Hicks and Anderson, *Women in Families,* p. 316.

Chapter VI

131 Uriel Halbreich . . . : Uriel Halbreich, M.D., "Hormones and Depression-0-Conceptual Transitions," *Hormones and Depression* (New York: Raven Press, 1987), p. 16.

133 Krohn quote: Faye Rice, "Menopause and the Working Woman," *Fortune,* Nov. 1994, pp. 203–6.

135 Researchers at the University of California . . . : Laurie Garrett, "The Estrogen Decision," *New York Newsday,* May 12, 1992.

135 Kronenberg quote: Fredi Kronenberg, Ph.D., spoke at a menopause workshop for the public in Kingston, New York, in 1993. The workshop was organized by medical writer Alice Goodman.

135 Dr. Philip M. Sarrel reported . . . : Lorna J. Sarrel, M.S.W., and Philip M. Sarrel, M.D., *Sexual Turning Points: The Seven Stages of Adult Sexuality* (New York: Macmillan, 1984), p. 257.

136 The cause of this sudden downward "resetting" . . . : Morris Notelovitz, M.D., Ph.D., and Diana Tonnessen, *Estrogen: Yes or No?* (New York: St. Martin's, 1993), p. 20. Dr. Notelovitz founded the Women's Medical and Diagnostic Center and Climacteric Clinic, in Gainesville, Florida, to provide medical care for pre- and postmenopausal women. Since 1980 he has supervised research and clinical management on more than 11,000 women age thirty and over, focusing on menopause.

136 Margaret Morganroth Gullette, "What, Menopause Again?" *Ms.,* July/ Aug. 1993, p. 34.

139 "This single hormonal change . . .": Sarrel and Sarrel, *Turning Points,* p. 265.

139 a number of symptoms can appear . . . : Ibid., p. 258.

139 "The loss of body control . . .": Ibid., p. 258.

140 Virtually all tissues . . . : Wulf H. Utian, M.D., Ph.D., speaking at "Menopause: Current Knowledge and Recommendations for Research," a conference sponsored by the National Institutes of Health, in

Bethesda, Maryland, March 22–24, 1993. Dr. Utian is honorary founding president and executive director, the North American Menopause Society; professor and chair of Reproductive Biology; Department of Obstetrics and Gynecology, Case Western Reserve University.

140 "urethral syndrome": Notelovitz and Tonnessen, *Estrogen: Yes or No?* p. 43.

141 Tavris quote: Carol Tavris, Ph.D., *The Mismeasure of Woman* (New York: Simon and Schuster, 1992), p. 150.

141 "enhances short-term memory . . .": Barbara Sherwin, Ph.D., in "Sex Hormones and Psychological Functioning," a talk presented at "Menopause: Current Knowledge and Recommendations for Research."

141 the number of words that women could recall . . . : Ibid.

142 "there was somewhat of an increase in score.": Ibid.

142 "a significant decrease": Ibid.

143 McEwen quotes: Bruce McEwen, Ph.D., "Effects of Estrogen and Neuronal Physiology and Architecture," presented at "Menopause: Current Knowledge and Recommendations for Research." McEwen is professor and head, Laboratory of Neuroendocrinology, Rockefeller University, New York City.

143 Catherine Wooley . . . : Ibid.

144 Kimura quote: Doreen Kimura, "How Sex Hormones Boost—or Cut—Intellectual Ability," *Psychology Today*, Nov. 1989, p. 63.

145 Tavris quote: *Psychology Today*, Nov. 1989.

145 Fausto-Sterling quote: Ibid., p. 62.

145 It was her studies documenting . . . : Diane L. Kampen, Ph.D., and Barbara B. Sherwin, Ph.D., "Estrogen Use and Verbal Memory in Healthy Postmenopausal Women," *Obstetrics and Gynecology*, vol. 83, no. 6 (June 1994), p. 979.

149 Douglas quote: Janice Douglas, M.D., "Cellular and Molecular Mechanisms of Estrogen Effects on Cardiovascular Function," presented at "Menopause: Current Knowledge and Recommendations for Research." Douglas is director, Division of Endocrinology and Hypertension, School of Medicine, University Hospitals of Cleveland, Case Western Reserve University.

149 The first inkling . . . : *The New England Journal of Medicine*, Sept. 12, 1991. Directed by Dr. Meier J. Stampfer of the Brigham and Women's Hospital in Boston, the study followed 48,470 menopausal women who were 30 to 64 years of age and who had no history of cancer or heart disease when the study began. The drawback of the nurses' study is that it could not provide definitive proof of estrogen's benefits because the participants were not randomly assigned to take estrogen or no hormones after menopause. Instead, the women made the choices themselves.

150 Douglas quote: Douglas, "Cellular and Molecular."

150 A 1990 study conducted in his clinic: Notelovitz and Tonnessen, *Estrogen: Yes or No?* p. 60.

150 "The plaque size is directly related . . .": Douglas, "Cellular and Molecular."

150 Among those who should seriously consider estrogen . . . : Notelovitz and Tonnessen, *Estrogen: Yes or No?* p. 66.

151 Brody quote: Jane Brody, "Hormone Replacement Study Answers Questions, But Not All," *The New York Times,* Jan. 18, 1995, p. C1.

151 Increasing evidence shows . . . : L. S. Richelson, L. J. Melton, et al., "Relative Contributions of Aging and Estrogen Deficiency to Postmenopausal Bone Loss," *New England Journal of Medicine,* vol. 311 (1984), pp. 1273–75.

151 Doress and Siegal quote: Paula Brown Doress and Diana Laskin Siegal, *Ourselves Growing Older* (New York: Simon and Schuster, 1987), p. 269.

152 Fully 50 percent of women . . . : Karen Westerberg Reyes, "Osteoporosis: The Silent Crippler," *Modern Maturity,* June/July 1993, p. 76.

152 Huppert quotes: Leonore C. Huppert, M.D., "Hormonal Replacement Therapy: Benefits, Risks, Doses," *Medical Clinics of North America,* vol. 71, no. 1 (Jan. 1989), p. 320.

152 women who think they can forget . . . : Quoted in Jane Brody, "Personal Health," *The New York Times,* July 14, 1993, p. C12.

153 The sooner hormone replacement is begun . . . : Huppert, "Hormonal Replacement Therapy," p. 27.

153 "When estrogen therapy is discontinued . . .": Ibid. Huppert is reporting results of a study by R. Lindsay, A. MacLean, and A. Kraszowski, et al., "Bone Response to Termination of Estrogen Treatment," *Lancet,* vol. 1 (1978), pp. 1325–29.

154 Among women who *do* have this history . . . : Notelovitz and Tonnessen, *Estrogen: Yes or No?* p. 96.

155 the risk of breast cancer . . . : "HRT and Breast Cancer Risk," *Harvard Women's Health Watch,* Aug. 1995, p. 1.

157 Over an 85-year life span . . . : Jane Brody, "Personal Health," *The New York Times,* Nov. 10, 1993, p. C17.

157 *risk of getting colon cancer:* "Estrogen vs. a Cancer," *The New York Times,* July 19, 1995, p. C3.

157 Dr. Huppert calls these conditions . . . : Huppert, "Hormonal Replacement Therapy."

157 Dr. Notelovitz adds to that list . . . : Notelovitz and Tonnessen, *Estrogen: Yes or No?* p. 101.

158 Parry quote: Barbara Parry, Ph.D., presented her research at a seminar, "Toward a New Psychobiology of Depression," at the 1992 meeting of the American Psychiatric Association in Washington, D.C. Parry has de-

voted much of her career to studying the biological correlates of depression. At the APA meeting she spoke about hormonal influences on mood disorders and reproductive events in women.

159 Weissman quote: Myrna Weissman, at "Toward a New Psychobiology of Depression."

159 Severino and Moline quote: Sally K. Severino, M.D., and Margaret L. Moline, Ph.D., *Premenstrual Syndrome* (New York: Guilford Press, 1989).

159 In a recent study of women taking estrogen . . . : Barbara B. Sherwin, "The Impact of Different Doses of Estrogen and Progestin on Mood and Sexual Behavior in Postmenopausal Women," *Journal of Clinical Endocrinology and Metabolism,* vol. 72, no. 2 (1991), p. 336.

160 Researchers in the United Kingdom . . . : C. B. Ballinger, M. C. Browning, and A. H. Smith, "Hormone Profiles and Psychological Symptoms in Peri-Menopausal Women," *Maturitas* (Nov. 1987).

162 Barbara Sherwin's lab . . . : Kampen and Sherwin, "Estrogen Use and Verbal Memory."

162 "Estrogen users recalled . . .": Kampen and Sherwin, "Estrogen Use and Verbal Memory."

162 Henderson quote: Philip H. Hilts, "Studies Suggest Estrogen Lowers Alzheimer's Risk," *The New York Times,* Nov. 10, 1993, p. A23.

162 Toran-Allerand quote: Natalie Angier, "How Estrogen May Work to Protect Against Alzheimer's," *The New York Times,* Mar. 8, 1994, p. C3.

163 "which extend from the body . . .": Ibid.

163 "That enzyme deficit . . .": Ibid.

163 "Neuroscientists have expressed . . .": Ibid.

164 Kimura quote: Doreen Kimura, "Sex Differences in the Brain."

164 Testosterone loss may also affect . . . : Natalie Angier, "A Male Menopause?" *The New York Times,* June 20, 1992, p. C14.

164 Hoberman and Yesalis quote: John M. Hoberman and Charles E. Yesalis, "The History of Synthetic Testosterone," *Scientific American,* Feb. 1995.

164 Angier quote: "Does Testosterone Equal Aggression? Maybe Not," *The New York Times,* June 20, 1995, p. 1.

166 "Indeed, aging is increasingly . . .": Ibid.

166 McKinlay quote: Angier, "A Male Menopause?"

167 60 percent of those who start . . . : Robert Rebar presented these statistics at "Menopause: Current Knowledge and Recommendations for Research." Dr. Rebar is professor and director of OB/GYN at the University of Cincinnati.

Chapter VII

170 Many women do report a lowered . . . : Ellen Cole, "Sex at Menopause: Each in Her Own Way," in *Women and Therapy*, ed. Ellen Cole and Esther Rosenblum (Binghamton, NY: Haworth Press, 1988), p. 163.

170 "It takes me fifteen minutes . . .": Ibid., p. 161.

171 Pomeroy quote: Carin Rubenstein, "The *Lear's* Report: How AIDS Has Changed Our Sex Lives," *Lear's*, Nov. 1992, pp. 62–67.

171 In a survey of 800 . . . : Lorna J. Sarrel, M.S.W., and Philip M. Sarrel, M.D., *Sexual Turning Points: The Seven Stages of Adult Sexuality* (New York: Macmillan, 1984), p. 261.

171 Older women also experience . . . : Winnifred Cutler, *Love Cycles: The Science of Intimacy* (New York: Villard, 1991), p. 191.

171 "My clitoris has become . . .": Cole, "Sex at Menopause," p. 163.

171 In Sarrel's London Menopause Study . . . : Sarrel and Sarrel, *Turning Points*, p. 264.

172 more likely to have a strong interest in sex: Ibid.

172 "safe sex, reduction of wrist . . .": M. J. Neuberger, "Thing," *The Village Voice*, June 14, 1992, p. 38.

172 "Now I can enjoy . . .": Cole, "Sex at Menopause," p. 163.

174 "the Sahara desert": Cole, "Sex at Menopause," p. 162.

174 . . . complained of vaginal dryness: Sarrel and Sarrel, *Turning Points*, p. 261.

174 As estrogen wanes . . . : Morris Notelovitz, M.D., Ph.D., and Diana Tonnessen, *Estrogen: Yes or No?* (New York: St. Martin's, 1993), p. 36.

174 Long periods of abstinence . . . : Sarrel and Sarrel, *Turning Points*, p. 261.

175 "I draw back from touch . . .": Cole, "Sex at Menopause," p. 162.

175 It isn't known for sure . . . : Sarrel and Sarrel, *Turning Points*, p. 260.

175 "I didn't like the way it felt . . .": Ibid., p. 260.

176 "My husband is patient . . .": Cole, "Sex at Menopause," p. 163.

176 "This avoids the psychological trauma . . .": "Atrophic Vaginitis," *Hot Flash*, vol. 5, no. 2 (Spring 1986), p. 3.

177 "Am I withholding from him . . .": Cole, "Sex at Menopause," p. 161.

178 One in two American women . . . : Cutler, *Love Cycles*, p. 71.

179 all women lose testosterone . . . : Barbara B. Sherwin, "Sex Hormones and Psychological Functioning," at NIH conference, "Workshop on Menopause: Current Knowledge and Recommendations for Research," held at the National Institutes of Health, in Bethesda, MD, on March 22, 1993. Dr. Sherwin is associate professor, Department of Psychology, McGill University, Montreal, Canada.

179 Sherwin quotes: Barbara B. Sherwin, "A Comparative Analysis of the Role of Androgen in Human Male and Female Sexual Behavior: Behav-

ioral Specificity, Critical Thresholds, and Sensitivity," *Psychobiology*, vol. 16, no. 4 (1988), pp. 416–25.

180 A gynecologist at Chelsea . . . : John M. Hoberman and Charles E. Yesalis, "The History of Synthetic Testosterone," *Scientific American*, Feb. 1995.

180 Greer quote: Germaine Greer, *The Change* (New York: Alfred A. Knopf, 1992), p. 177.

183 After 45, most women experience . . . : Cutler, *Love Cycles*, p. 203.

184 Cutler quote: Ibid., p. 205.

184 Dr. Arnold Kegel . . . : Ibid., p. 204.

184 "To locate the circumvaginal muscle . . .": Notelovitz and Tonnessen, *Estrogen: Yes or No?* p. 54.

184 Feedback from the perineometer . . . : Cutler, *Love Cycles*, pp. 203–6.

185 Notelovitz quote: Notelovitz and Tonnessen, *Estrogen: Yes or No?* p. 55.

185 Iddenden quote: David Iddenden, "Sexuality During Menopause," *Medical Clinics of North America*, vol. 71, no. 1 (Jan. 1987), p. 91.

185 In a study conducted at Stanford . . . : Cutler, *Love Cycles*, p. 191.

185 At sixty, most men . . . : Jon Hendricks and C. Davis Hendricks, *Aging in Mass Society: Myths and Realities*, 3rd ed. (Boston: Little, Brown & Co., 1986), p. 274.

186 Scarf quote: Maggie Scarf, "The Middle of the Journey," *Family Therapy Networker*, July/Aug. 1992.

186 "The teenage male . . . The male nearing sixty . . .": Ibid.

187 Not surprisingly, men . . . : Cutler, *Love Cycles*, p. 116.

187 men with low testosterone . . . : Ibid., p. 112.

187 Besides testosterone therapy . . . : Ibid., p. 149.

187 One college professor . . . : Paul Delaney, "When Medication Affects Sex, Some Men Risk Hypertension," *The New York Times*, July 8, 1992, p. C12.

187 "Middle-age men who exercise . . .": Cutler, *Love Cycles*, p. 48.

188 In another study, 48-year-old men . . . : Mary Jo Schnatter, "Did You Know?" *McCall's*, Apr. 1992, p. 38.

188 One reason for the increase . . . : Sandra Blakeslee, "New Therapies Are Helping Men to Overcome Impotence," *The New York Times*, June 2, 1993.

188 The young adult male . . . : Scarf, "Middle of the Journey."

188 In 1992, neuroscientist . . . : Blakeslee, "New Therapies."

189 Smoking . . . : Ibid.

189 Other medical conditions . . . : Iddenden, "Sexuality During Menopause," p. 92.

189 Scarf quote: Scarf, "Middle of the Journey."

190 Cole quote: Cole, "Sex at Menopause," p. 10.

192 "As a woman coming to terms . . .": Rubenstein, "The *Lear's* Report."

192 In 1982, just 12 percent . . . : Deborah Kutzko, "Teaching Safe Sex to Women in the Age of AIDS," *Women and Therapy*, vol. 7, nos. 2 and 3 (1988), p. 71.

192 Catania quote: "Study Finds Many Heterosexuals Are Ignoring Serious Risk of AIDS," *The New York Times*, Nov. 13, 1992, p. A16.

192 Leslie quote: Norma J. Leslie, "Divorced Women's Sexual and Contraceptive Issues," *Women and Therapy*, vol. 7, nos. 2 and 3 (1988), pp. 269 and 266.

193 "can serve temporarily . . .": Ibid., p. 274.

195 Pudney quote: "HIV Cl   Supports Early Use of Condom," *The New York Times*, Dec. 8, 1992.

195 Oral sex . . . : Deborah Kutzko, "Teaching Safe Sex to Women in the Age of AIDS," *Women and Therapy*, ed. Cole and Rothulum, vol. 7, no. 2, Feb. 3, 1988.

196 Nearly one in four . . . : Rubinstein, *The Lears Report*, pp. 62–67.

196 "The only safe sex . . .": Ibid.

197 "Two years of celibacy . . .": Henie Lorant, "The Price of Protection," *The Woodstock Times*, Dec. 12, 1991, p. 32.

Chapter VIII

200 Anderson quote: Sharon Hicks and Carol M. Anderson, "Women on Their Own," in *Women in Families*, ed. Monica McGoldrick, Carol M. Anderson, and Froma Walsh (New York: W. W. Norton & Co., 1991), p. 37.

201 Jones-Lee quote: Anita Jones-Lee, *Women and Money* (Hauppauge, NY: Barron's, 1991), p. 5.

201 Lewis quote: Robert Lewis, "Equity Eludes Women," *AARP Bulletin*, Nov. 1991, pp. 1, 10–12.

201 A woman who's earning . . . : Maggie Mahar, "The Truth About Women's Pay," *Working Woman*, Apr. 1993.

201 In *Women and Money* . . . : Jones-Lee, *Women and Money*, p. 4.

201 men's stock portfolios . . . : Allen R. Myerson, "Wall Street Addresses Women's Distinct Needs," *The New York Times*, July 31, 1993.

201 A Merrill Lynch study . . . : Laurie Baum, "Corporate Women," *Business Week*, June 22, 1987, pp. 72–78.

202 In 1976, *Business Week* . . . : Ibid.

202 From proxy statements . . . : Jaclyn Fierman, "Why Women Still Don't Hit the Top," *Fortune*, July 30, 1990, pp. 40–62.

202 In a study published in 1995 . . . : Diana Bilimoria and Sandy Kristin Piderit, "Sexism on High: Corporate Boards," *The New York Times*, Feb. 5, 1995, p. F11.

203 In her peak year . . . : Meryl Gordon, "Discrimination at the Top," *Working Woman,* Sept. 1992, p. 68.

203 "I was very upset . . .": Ibid., p. 70.

204 *Business Week* quote: Baum, "Corporate Women," p. 72.

204 Golden quote: Ibid.

204 Only 20 percent of the husbands . . . : Arlie Hochschild, *The Second Shift: Working Parents and the Revolution at Home* (New York: Viking, 1989).

205 This extra work prevents . . . : Robyn I. Stone, "The Feminization of Poverty Among the Elderly," *Women's Studies Quarterly,* vol. 17 (Spring-Summer 1989), pp. 20–34.

205 To get an idea . . . : Jones-Lee, *Women and Money,* p. 7.

205 Built into the system . . . : Beth Hess, "Aging and Old Women: The Hidden Agenda," in *Gender and the Life Course,* ed. Alice S. Rossi (New York: Aldine, 1985), pp. 319–31.

205 Eighty percent . . . : Jane Seskin, "Alone But Not Lonely," *AARP Bulletin* (1985), p. 134.

206 Women's lifetime earnings . . . : Jones-Lee, *Women and Money,* p. 8.

206 Annually they receive . . . : National Organization for Women statistic, cited in Annette Lieberman and Vicki Lindner, *Unbalanced Accounts* (New York: Viking Penguin, 1988), p. 179.

206 Over the age of 65 . . . : Stone, "Feminization of Poverty."

208 Only 12.5 percent own stock . . . : Jones-Lee, *Women and Money,* p. 4.

208 Eighty percent of widowed women . . . : Lieberman and Lindner, *Unbalanced Accounts,* p. 144.

213 A California study . . . : Judith S. Wallerstein, Ph.D., "Women After Divorce: Preliminary Report from a Ten-Year Follow-up," *American Journal of Orthopsychiatry,* vol. 56 (Jan. 1986), p. 65.

213 Ten years after divorce . . . : Ibid., p. 73.

213 By the time they're of retirement age . . . : Namkee G. Choi, "Correlates of the Economic Status of Widowed and Divorced Elderly Women," *Journal of Family Issues,* vol. 13, no. 1 (Mar. 1992), p. 48.

213 Kirkpatrick quote: Martha Kirkpatrick, M.D., "Some Clinical Perceptions of Middle-Aged Divorced Women," in *Divorce as a Developmental Process,* ed. Judith Gold, M.D. (Washington, D.C.: American Psychiatric Press, 1988).

213 Spousal support . . . : Ibid.

213 Almost one in five . . . : Ibid.

213 Career assets . . . : Ibid.

213 Only 20 percent . . . : Diane P. Holder and Carol M. Anderson, "Women, Work, and the Family," in *Women in Families,* ed. McGoldrick, Anderson, and Walsh, p. 376.

214 Whether they are single . . . : Rosalind C. Barnett, "Women in Man-

agement Today," Center for Research on Women, no. 249 (Wellesley, MA: Wellesley College, 1992), p. 21.

214 Lieberman and Lindner quote: Lieberman and Lindner, *Unbalanced Accounts*, p. 127.

214 "She's wearing black and pearls . . .": Ibid., p. 130.

215 Fear of ending up destitute . . . : Ibid.

216 Women who reject . . . : Ibid., p. 229.

222 "If a woman invests five thousand dollars . . .": Myerson, "Wall Street Addresses."

224 Surveys show that women are more likely . . . : Ibid.

224 "They tend to put less of their money . . .": Ibid.

224 "No matter what I do with money . . .": Ann Conover Heller, "How to Make Money by Risking It," *Lear's*, Sept. 1991, p. 77.

CHAPTER IX

230 The shift from early adulthood . . . : Bertram J. Cohler, "Personal Narrative and the Life Course" in *Life-Span Development and Behavior*, eds. Paul B. Baltes and Orville G. Brim, Jr., vol. 4 (New York: Academic Press, 1982), p. 215.

231 Mason quote: Marilyn Mason, "The Wilderness Within: Feminist Guide to Adult Development," presented at the Fiftieth Anniversary Conference of the American Association for Marriage and Family Therapy, in Miami in 1992.

233 Nef quotes: Lydia Bronte, *The Longevity Factor* (New York: HarperCollins, 1993), pp. 215–17.

235 Psychologist Dean Keith Simonton . . . : Ibid., p. 49.

235 Bronte quote: Ibid., p. 16.

242 Conley quote: Jane Gross, "A Woman's Quitting Touches Nerve at Medical School," *The New York Times*, July 14, 1991, Section I, Part I, p. 10.

247 Heilbrun quote: Carolyn Heilbrun, *Writing a Woman's Life* (New York: Ballantine Books, 1988), p. 44.

248 People are constantly weaving . . . : Bernice L. Neugarten, "Interpretive Social Science and Research on Aging," *Gender and the Life Course*, ed. Alice S. Rossi (New York: Aldine, 1985), p. 298.

248 "they will not . . .": Heilbrun, *Writing*, p. 46.

251 "The inner life of the mind . . .": Bernice L. Neugarten, "Time, Age, and the Life Cycle," *The American Journal of Psychiatry*, vol. 136, no. 7 (July 1979), p. 893.

253 Heilbrun quote: Heilbrun, *Writing*, p. 126.

INDEX

Women's movement, 3, 7–8
Woodman, Marion, 64–66, 67, 105
Wooley, Catherine, 143
Work issues, 55, 77–78
  and menopause, 132
  See also Double day; Glass ceiling; Income, women's; Pensions
Working Woman (magazine), 34, 203
Wylie, Philip, 84, 86

Y

Yale Menopause Clinic, 90, 139, 170, 174, 177
Yaskin, Judith, 114
Yesalis, Charles E., 164, 180
Youthfulness, 28, 79–83

Z

Zacher, Millicent, 189

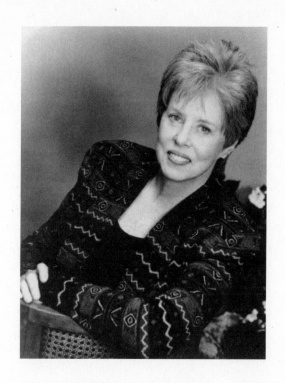

About the Author

COLETTE DOWLING is the author of the million-copy-plus best-seller *The Cinderella Complex, You Mean I Don't Have to Feel This Way?,* and *Perfect Women.* She lectures nationwide, and more than 100 of her articles have appeared in major magazines. The mother of three grown children, she lives in New York City and Woodstock.